The Nurse's Guide *to* Medicines

The Nurse's Guide *to* Medicines

Sheila Cunningham *and* Rachael Major

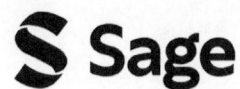

S Sage

1 Oliver's Yard
55 City Road
London EC1Y 1SP

2455 Teller Road
Thousand Oaks, California 91320

Unit No 323-333, Third Floor, F-Block
International Trade Tower Nehru Place
New Delhi 110 019

8 Marina View Suite 43-053
Asia Square Tower 1
Singapore 018960

Editor: Laura Walmsley
Editorial Assistant: Sahar Jamfar
Production Editor: Gourav Kumar
Copyeditor: Tom Bedford
Proofreader: Sarah Cooke
Indexer: Cathryn Pritchard
Marketing Manager: Ruslana Khatagova
Cover Design: Sheila Tong
Typeset by KnowledgeWorks Global Ltd
Printed in the UK

Library of Congress Control Number: 2023952317

British Library Cataloguing in Publication data

A catalogue record for this book is available from the British Library

ISBN 978-1-5296-0383-5
ISBN 978-1-5296-0382-8 (pbk)

CONTENTS

ABOUT THE AUTHORS

Sheila Cunningham commenced her career as a nurse after which she undertook a BSc in Life Sciences (Human Physiology) at Westminster University. Armed with this and a passion for all things physiology, pathology and pharmacology she taught on nursing and allied health profession programmes for many years and explored pedagogical approaches aimed at improving and enhancing nurses' knowledge and confidence with science for clinical practice. Through her doctoral work on inclusive learning she linked her teaching and subject knowledge especially around nurse and health professions education. She was programme lead for Nursing Exchange and the BSc in European Nursing until 2020, hence her interest in nursing international experiences. She holds a National Teaching Fellowship and is a member of the Biosciences in Nursing Network (BiNE). She is currently Deputy Dean for Research and Knowledge Exchange in the Faculty of Health Social Care and Education at Middlesex University.

Rachael Major completed a BSc (Hons) in Physiology at University College London before starting nursing. Over many years of teaching, she has used that degree to pass on her knowledge and passion for all biological sciences to many nursing and healthcare students, leading on modules across all three years of the nursing degree programme and at postgraduate level. During her Masters in Higher Education she researched the teaching of biological sciences to nursing students and her doctoral and post-doctoral work on dyslexia and neurodiversity in nursing has influence how she supports students' learning. She is a member of BiNE and is a Senior Fellow of AdvanceHE. She is currently the Postgraduate Programmes and Academic CPD Lead and Equality, Diversity and Inclusion Lead at the Institute of Health and Social Care Studies in Guernsey.

ACKNOWLEDGEMENTS

Thank you to all our nursing and midwifery teaching colleagues and clinical staff with whom we have the pleasure to work. In addition thanks goes to all our students in undergraduate and postgraduate study who we strive to support in becoming the best professionals of the future.

Sheila Cunningham and Rachael Major

INTRODUCTION

We are pleased to present this book, *The Nurse's Guide to Medicines*, for adult nursing and healthcare students and newly qualified nurses to provide a simple and easy-to-read guide to frequently used medicines in adult patient settings.

Nurses play an integral role in administering medication to patients, and depending on the environment in which they work this could be as often as every few minutes. A good understanding of pharmacology is therefore essential to the safe administration of medications. Advanced skills and roles of nurses such as prescribing require nurses to be well prepared and informed. This also includes knowledge of medicines and actions as well as medicines optimisation and clinical decision making. As such nurses need to keep their knowledge refreshed and up to date from pre-qualification onwards throughout their careers. This book aims to support this by expanding and consolidating this knowledge and application.

This book adopts a conceptual learning approach where medicines and pharmacology are not abstract 'science' but integrated into patient care. This supports students and nurses to develop and improve critical thinking, enhances their self-efficacy and ultimately professional practice. This is particularly useful if nurses are to think about or engage with prescribing relatively soon after qualification. It must be noted that this book is not intended as a 'prescriber's guide' nor is it intended to replace formal regulated guidance on medicines, doses and prescribing. It is intended as a reference guide and information and as a learning tool. It is highly recommended that medical and pharmaceutical advice is sought, such as from the British National Formulary (JFC 2023), alongside local policies, guidance and relevant legislation and professional codes and scope of practice.

The authors of this book are registered nurses and nurse teachers. They both have bachelor's degrees in bioscience-related subjects, teaching qualifications and have taught biosciences and pharmacology for many years. All case studies used within this book are based and adapted from real clinical experiences anonymised to maintain confidentiality and anonymity.

The aim of this book is to provide a simple easy-to-read guide to either refresh knowledge or to provide a platform for further exploration of more complex pharmacological texts and research into medications. The conceptual approach supports the complex nature of patients, and the subsequent medication regimes reflecting the multiple and complex health conditions of the UK population today (CoDH, 2016). Medicines are part of a 'care approach' and as such are proposed to be seen as integral to the complex patient situation and needs.

This book is suitable for a wide range of healthcare professionals, both students and practitioners, but is written primarily with students (nurses, nursing associates etc.) in mind. It is also suitable for those carers in a wide variety of care settings who wish to understand more about medication and types.

There are nine chapters in total. Each chapter is written in a specific format to enable the reader to see the core features at a glance and then specific content moves from simple to more complex and applied aspects at the end. Each chapter will begin with clear objectives detailing what the reader will achieve. It will have an overview and the rationale of the medicine area then present key medications in summarised form. Each chapter will incorporate a case study and prompt questions to apply and consolidate the learning, answers to the case study, a chapter summary and recommended reading and resources. A glossary at the end of the book will provide explanation and clarity on terminology used within the book.

There is some expected knowledge required to approach this book and obtain the full benefit. The nurse or healthcare professional is recommended to be familiar with key terminology and processes (outlined below). Whilst some fundamental knowledge is expected it is acknowledged that with increasing advances in drug types, routes and personalised medicines etc. this terminology is ever expanding. Some terminology such as drug or medicine is used interchangeably; the key difference is the chemical product (drug) and the application to treat a condition or exert a biological effect (medicine). A brief reminder of the key terms and processes is summarised below. This is not exhaustive, but a brief reminder:

Terminology	Meaning
Pharmacology	The scientific study of drugs and their effects on living systems.
Pharmacokinetics	The measurement and interpretation of the changes over time of drug concentrations in differing parts of the body: absorption, distribution, metabolism, excretion. Also colloquially known as 'what the body does to the drug'.
Pharmacodynamics	The interaction of the drug with the body tissues, how it exerts its cellular or tissue effect. Also colloquially known as 'what the drug does to the body'.
Pharmacovigilance	The science and activities relating to the detection, assessment, understanding and prevention of adverse effects or any other medicine-related problem.
Pharmacosurveillance	Refers to the monitoring of drugs once they reach the market after clinical trials. That is when they are used on patients/people. This is the means to detect previously unrecognised positive or negative effects that may be associated with a drug. The majority of postmarketing surveillance concerns adverse drug reactions monitoring and evaluation. Suspected adverse drug reactions can be directly reported to the Medicines and Healthcare products Regulatory Agency (MHRA) through the Yellow Card Scheme using the electronic form at www.mhra.gov.uk/yellowcard
Pharmacogenetics	Refers to the study of genetic causes of individual variations in drug response.

Pharmacogenomics	Concerns the impact of multiple gene mutations (genome) that might determine a patient's response to drug therapy.
Pharmacoepidemiology	This is the study of drugs in large populations and the effects. It could be termed a type of pharmacovigilance.
Pharmacoeconomics	This concerns the costs of medicines and comparing across differing drugs.
Psychopharmacology	The study of how drugs affect the brain and behaviour. May also be connected to drugs for treating mental health conditions.
Pharmacy	This refers to the process, person and place involved in preparing and dispensing prescription drugs and is a healthcare resource in the community.
Drug licensing	Multiple elements to this – it falls under legislation to address general licensing, personal licensing and costs to pharmaceutical companies for holding licenses – see: www.gov.uk/government/collections/drugs-licensing
Adverse drug reaction (ADR)	Also known as *adverse effects* or *side effects* but best described as ADR. It is a response to a medicinal product, or combination of medicinal products, which is noxious and unintended (MHRA, 2015). There are different categories of ADR (do refer to MHRA, 2015). The terms 'adverse reaction' and 'adverse effect' are interchangeable but reflect different points of view: a drug has an adverse effect, whereas a person experiences an adverse reaction.
Therapeutic drugs	Broadly is a group of drugs categorised from a medical perspective by the pathology they are used to treat, e.g. antibiotics, anti-inflammatories, stimulant.

All are important, but for this book the key terms to keep in mind are **pharmacokinetics**, **pharmacodynamics**, **pharmacovigilance**.

We hope that you enjoy the book and find it useful.

REFERENCES

Council of Deans for Health (CoDH) (2016) Educating the future nurse – a paper for discussion. https://councilofdeans.org.uk/wp-content/uploads/2016/08/Educating-the-Future-Nurse-FINAL-1.pdf

Joint Formulary Committee (2023) British National Formulary (online) London: BMJ and Pharmaceutical Press http://www.medicinescomplete.com [Accessed on 20/02/2024]

Medicines and Healthcare Regulatory Authority (MHRA) (2015) Guidance on adverse drug reactions. Medicines and Healthcare Products Regulatory Agency. https://assets. publishing.service.gov.uk/government/uploads/system/uploads/attachment_data/ file/949130/Guidance_on_adverse_drug_reactions.pdf

1 MEDICINES OPTIMISATION AND MANAGEMENT

SHEILA CUNNINGHAM

AFTER READING THIS CHAPTER YOU WILL BE ABLE TO:

- Differentiate between medicines management and medicines optimisation.
- Discuss the importance of understanding the patient experience to improve adherence to medicines regimes.
- Describe and argue the rationale for 'evidence-based choice of medicines'.
- Explain the nurse's role in medicines safety for patients.

WHAT IS MEDICINES OPTIMISATION OR MANAGEMENT?

Nurses will come across medicines in all areas of patient care since they are a most common intervention in healthcare for the prevention, treatment and/or management of many illnesses (JFC, 2022; National Institute for Health and Care Excellence (NICE), 2015). As the population ages and illnesses become more complex (multi-morbidities) there will be an increasing need for more medicines with potentially confusing or complicated medication regimes. Alongside this, the availability and use of prescribed medicines can be confounded further if mixed with other sources of medicines, i.e. over-the-counter (OTC) medicines or nutritional supplements. Consequently, patient treatment may be affected and potentially lead to an increased risk to patients in the longer term. NICE (2024) report that approximately 33% to 50% of medicines prescribed for long-term conditions are not taken as intended, or if started well are not taken consistently or continued. It appears 5 to 8% of hospital admissions are a consequence of ineffective or inappropriate use of medicines and up to 6.5% result from adverse effects of medicines (Kaufman 2015). One Cochrane evidence review reported that many people who are prescribed medication to self-administer only take half of their prescribed dose, and many cease their medication entirely or do not take it in the way it is prescribed without informing their prescriber (Nieuwlaat et al., 2014). This issue of non-adherence to medicines may for a number of reasons either be intentional or unintentional or a combination of both. This will certainly interfere with the intended aims of treatment and create or contribute to longer-term problems.

Nurses (students, qualified and nursing associates) are highly visible in all aspects of patient care and so are ideally situated to guide, clarify and support patients with their medicines. The NMC (2018) nurse education proficiencies outline the knowledge required of pharmacology and an understanding of medicines management (Platform 4 and Annexe 5) applied to practice. As such medicines and treatments are integral to person-centred care and form part of care planning and reviewing. Nurses, therefore, need to possess accurate knowledge not just of the medication and indications. This does not mean memorising them (this would be impossible) but possess the skills to research and evaluate them in reputable texts and sources (such as the British National Formulary). Additionally, nurses need to be conscious of patient behaviours and attitudes around taking medications to ensure optimal effects. As in all care planning this requires assessing the problem, planning, implementing, evaluating and reviewing care (and medicines) in an iterative cycle by the care team. This may necessitate regular review and identifying issues patients' hold regarding 'adhering' to prescribed medications or challenges they may encounter.

WATCH OUT!

Medicines optimisation priorities (based on NICE, 2015):

- Patient safety reporting using established processes for adverse drug incidents
- Medicine review
- Medicines reconciliation
- Patient as a partner in decision making around medicines
- Clear and open communication and consistency of medicines for patients moving settings (hospital or home)

Medicines optimisation is the currently accepted term (NICE, 2015) for helping patients get the best outcome from their medicines. It is a shift to a humanised patient-centred approach for medicines focusing on how patients use medicines over time. This may mean stopping some medicines or starting or changing others whilst also considering opportunities for other interventions (non-medicine), for example lifestyle changes to reduce the need for medicines (RPS, 2013). One example to illustrate this may be a person with hypertension who, in ongoing review, does not require a prescription of anti-hypertensive medicines since, through lifestyle changes, they lost weight and have a regular exercise regimen which manages their hypertension.

This holistic approach to medicines involves the wider healthcare team (including pharmacists, prescribers and nurses). This reflects an integrated care and partnership approach around medicines as patient care practice. Medicines optimisation is a major concern. The NHS spent a total of £17.1 billion in 2020/21, an increase of 4.56% from the £16.4 billion in 2019/20 – this is the second-highest area of spending in the NHS, after staffing costs (NHSBA, 2022). Medicines also have the potential to cause harm. Between 5 and 10% of all hospital admissions are medicines-related, two-thirds of medicines-related hospital admissions are preventable and 30–50% of medicines prescribed for long-term conditions are not taken as intended (NHS, 2015).

Medicines reconciliation is another related concept. It is defined as the process of identifying an accurate list of medicines a person is taking including all prescribed and acquired from various sources such as over the counter medicines and comparing them with the current list in use by the prescriber/physician, recognising any discrepancies, and documenting any changes, thereby resulting in a complete list of medicines, accurately communicated (NICE, 2016). It is worth noting the term 'medicines' extends beyond those prescribed by a physician or prescriber. It also includes OTC, supplementary and complementary medicines or herbs. There is a section in the British National Formulary which outlines the main complementary and herbal preparations in use and any effects on other conventional medicines. However this group comprises a broad range so the principles mentioned above support assessments and decisions to optimise medicines taking.

Two key documents which are most useful around these issues are the NICE quality standard on medicines optimisation (QS120; 2016) and the NICE clinical guidelines on medicines adherence (2009, reviewed 2019). Whilst several terms have been introduced so far, there are others within the literature with connected but different meanings, and will be beneficial to your understanding to read these over; they are presented in the box below.

DEFINITIONS CONNECTED TO MEDICINES OPTIMISATION

Medicines management: 'system of processes and behaviours that determine how medicines are used by the NHS and patients' (NICE, 2015).

Medicine adherence: 'The process by which patients take their medications as prescribed, composed of initiation, implementation and discontinuation. Initiation occurs when the patient takes the first dose of a prescribed medication' (Vrijens et al., 2012).

Medicines optimisation: 'a person centred approach to safe and effective medicines use, to ensure people obtain the best possible outcomes from their medicine' (NICE, 2015).

Medicines concordance: 'is an older more complicated term which describes an approach to the prescribing and taking of medicines as an 'agreement' between a patient and a healthcare professional that respects the beliefs and wishes of the patient in determining whether, when and how medicines are to be taken. Whilst often a synonym for optimisation it should be emphasised that does not mean the same thing' (NCCSDO, 2005).

Medicine compliance: 'a relationship in which the role of the clinician is to decide on the appropriate treatment and issue the relevant instructions, whereas the role of the patient is to passively follow 'the doctor's orders' (NCCSDO, 2005).

Medicines optimisation addresses the following:

- Review of medicines (use and effect)
- Effect of polypharmacy (multiple medicines)
- Communication, guidance and support in relation to medicines
- The use of processes such as: deprescribing; medicines reconciliation, reviews and repeat prescribing; problematic polypharmacy
- Reducing medication waste and errors
- Self-management plans (RCN and RPS, 2020; BNF, 2022).

Central to this is patient experience which includes the practicalities of accessing and taking medicines as well as their attitudes and beliefs towards medicines. Medicines are chemicals and are prescribed to effect a physiological change, either to replace or control some function or symptom. However, the patient is not a passive recipient – they have their own behaviours and views and this has the potential to impact the therapeutic aim and pharmacological actions. This might include altered patterns of administration, ingestion or timing resulting in ineffective or excessive blood levels or distribution (pharmacokinetics) or ineffective action or excess action at tissues (pharmacodynamic). Readers are reminded to consult a good-quality pharmacology text to refresh their memories on these terms if they need to. The consequences could be serious or less so. These include unacceptable adverse effects or creating other physiological problems with the serious potential of being misunderstood as another condition. Further consequences could also be ineffectiveness, or worse, compromised patient safety.

NURSE'S ROLE IN MEDICINES OPTIMISATION

The World Health Organisation (2017) asserts that people are not always 'medication-wise'. In all encounters with patients, nurses and other healthcare professionals have an opportunity to evaluate a patient's situation, and understand and evaluate their relationship with medicines. Patients with chronic conditions have been reported to experience considerable issues with medications (multiple medications, drug interactions, adherence issues etc.) and having a clear overview and acting as an advocate and guide are recommended (RCN and RPS, 2020). Vulnerable groups such as the elderly, those who are confused or unable to make decisions or in the most socio-economically deprived groups are definitely in need of advocacy. These patients are more likely to have long-term conditions with increased severity (Kings Fund, n.d.). Ultimately communication and patient care episodes provide ample opportunities for addressing issues with medicines such as administration, palatability, route, timing, food and duration.

A fundamental knowledge and awareness by nurses and healthcare professionals is required of medicine side effects, recommended doses and dosing regimens for optimum effects. Simultaneously it is necessary to be mindful of drug interactions or side effects which may require other medicines to manage them. For example, a patient taking medicines for pain such as arthritis may take a mix of specific and non specific pain relief (e.g. ibuprofen) or steroids, and the common effect of these is gastric irritation which requires further medicine for relief. Or if patients are taking stronger pain relief medicines such as codeine phosphate these may lead to serious side effects which need other medication such as for nausea, constipation or drowsiness. This could potentially lead to a serious patient safety concern (falls, trips) as well as a need to manage the adverse effects.

MEDICINES ADHERENCE: INTENTIONAL OR NON-INTENTIONAL NON-ADHERENCE

Medication adherence refers to the extent to which medication taking corresponds with agreed recommendations from a healthcare professional and prescriber. Medication non-adherence can be classified as intentional or unintentional according to the patient's perspective or behaviours, and is a worldwide concern (WHO, 2017).

- Intentional non-adherence is where patients make a deliberate decision not to follow the prescribed medication regimen, such as altering the dose, timing or frequency of their medicine therapy. Furthermore, patients' beliefs about their pathology or condition and medication may also influence non-adherence.
- Unintentional non-adherence includes behaviours such as forgetting to use the medication. This may be especially prevalent when the patient has been using their medication for an extended period.

Non-adherence may be mistaken for treatment failure if not investigated specifically. A relatively recent study (de Jager et al., 2018) found that non-adherence rather than poor response to treatment was the cause of poor control of hypertension in 35% of people. Therefore, healthcare professionals should consider non-adherence to be a significant factor in treatment failure and should attempt to discuss this with the person before any further medicines are prescribed. Failure to address this may lead to more medicines being prescribed, potentially increasing the risks associated with polypharmacy, which in turn may cause harm to the person without the underlying illness being effectively treated.

MEDICINES OPTIMISATION AND MEDICATION SAFETY IN POLYPHARMACY

The challenges faced around polypharmacy are inextricably linked to the fact that as the number of medicines prescribed increases, the risk from adverse effects increases too. Medication safety is a particular concern in key groups, such as older people, and medicines optimisation also includes safety issues such as adverse drug reactions (ADRs) – unwanted effects or harmful reactions experienced by the patient whilst taking the medication prescribed. ADRs account for around 6.5% (Osanlou et al., 2022) to 8% (Insani et al., 2021) of hospital admissions, with approximately 70% of these ADRs deemed avoidable. There is an established mechanism for reporting ADRs and each report is collated, investigated and analysed; this is known as the 'Yellow Card Scheme' managed by the Medicines and Healthcare Products Regulatory Agency (MHRA). This scheme is voluntary, though all healthcare professionals and patients are encouraged to use it if there are ADRs. It can be found in the British National Formulary (BNF) hard copy or online. These reports are welcomed for the ongoing monitoring of drug reactions, however they do not always indicate the cause or that one adverse reaction may be due to another medicine being taken at the same time, or a complication of polypharmacy. Whilst the Yellow Card Scheme is important for prescribed drugs it is also useful for non-prescribed medicines such as OTC or those purchased over the internet – a phenomenon which surged during the Covid-19 pandemic. The Government urges caution with obtaining medicines on the internet because of risks due to lack of supervision of a healthcare professional and the potential risk from the medicine which could be out of date, counterfeit or diluted (See #FakeMeds campaign 2022 run by the MHRA).

GO FURTHER

ADRs: Reporting (https://yellowcard.mhra.gov.uk/)
    What is considered suitable to report? The MHRA indicate:

- All reactions to medicines which require 'additional monitoring' (i.e. drugs marked with inverted black triangle ▼) since they are newer with less established adverse effects.
- Any suspected serious reaction to all other medicines:
  - Prescription medicines
  - OTC medications
  - Herbal medicines
  - Vaccines
  - Blood products
  - Dental and surgical materials
  - Fake medicines or medical devices
  - Side effects or safety concerns about e-cigarettes

Over 50% of medication errors occur in four drug classes: antiplatelets, non-steroidal anti-inflammatory drugs (NSAIDs), diuretics and anticoagulants. Use of medicines which are not prescribed (i.e. over-the-counter medicines from pharmacies, herbal preparations, supplements or even someone's else's prescription drugs such as pain relief) also link to increased unwanted adverse effects or treatment concerns. Medicines most likely to be related to a hospital admission include the following:

- Antiplatelets (Chapter 6)
- NSAIDs (Chapter 7)
- Diuretics (Chapter 4)
- Anticoagulants (Chapter 6)
- Angiotensin converting enzyme (ACE) inhibitors (Chapter 6)

The above are addressed within other chapters and will not be included here. Other products or food substances to consider for unwanted and adverse effects include the examples below; whilst not 'drugs' they are included in the BNF under 'drugs' but acknowledged as food substances with significant effects. These will form the medicine 'monographs' of information here:

- St John's Wort
- Grapefruit juice
- Cranberry juice

NICE (2015) urge the need for evidence-based use of medicines and prescribing or reviewing of medicines for patient safety. This then is a foundation for working through the next chapters in this book addressing specific medicine groups and related interactions or dose considerations.

Drug (herb) name: St John's Wort

UK brand names: St John's Wort is a herbal medicine with a wide range of properties affecting serotonin levels. It is not approved for use as a medicine but is widely available in health food and other shops as a herbal supplement. It is included only for its potential to interact with drugs.

Average doses:

- Two 300 mg tablets once daily (depending on brand and formulation)

What form does it come in: Tablet, capsule, tincture, teabags

Does it interact with other medicines: Yes, over 244 interactions reported in BNF (2022). The following serious interactions are known:

- Results in decreased effectiveness of:
    o Cancer treatments: Abemaciclib, Acalabrutinib, Avapritinib, Irinotecan, Cabazitaxel
    o Cardiac/rhythmic drugs: Dronedarone
    o Anticoagulants: acenocoumarol, apixaban
    o Aminophylline
    o Antivirals: Atazanavir, Darunavir, Imatinib, Dasatinib
    o Graft rejection blockers: cyclosporin and tacrolimus
    o Anti-tuberculosis: Bedaquiline
    o Chronic kidney disease: Finerenone
    o Benzodiazepines: Midazolam
    o Opioids: Methadone, Oxycodone
    o HIV treatment: Nevirapine
    o Contraceptive hormones: Norethisterone, Levonorgestrel
    o Anti-seizure: phenobarbital, phenytoin.
- Alter serotonin levels and risk of serotonin syndrome:
    o Antidepressant medication: escitalopram, amitriptyline, Phenelizine
    o Antiemetics: Ondansetron, Granisetron
    o Analgesia: Pentazocine.
- Increased risk of severe hypotension: anaesthetic agents, e.g. Digoxin, Desflurane.
- Increased efficacy of metabolic medication inhibitor of glucosylceramide synthase: Eliglustat.

Caution: St John's Wort is unlicensed and self-administered so taking this may not recorded and needs to be part of patient assessment.

(Continued)

Drug (food substance) name: Grapefruit juice

UK brand names: Grapefruit juice is a food substance included only for its potential to interact with drug metabolism.

Average doses:

- There is no average amount – this is self-consumed

What form does it come in: Liquid and solid (fruit) form

Does it interact with other medicines: Yes, several. Some of the following interactions are known:

- Increase drug availability and effect of:
    - Simvastin (Statins)
    - Calcium channel blockers:
        - Amlodipine
        - Felodipine
        - Lacidipine
        - Lercanidipine
        - Nicardipine
        - Nifedipine
        - Nimodipine
        - Verapamil
    - Warfarin (Anticoagulant)
    - Anti-platelet (increases circulating drug):
        - Clopidogrel
        - Ticagrelor
    - Glucocorticoid: Budesonide
    - Graft rejection blockers: Cyclosporin and tacrolimus.

Drug (food substance) name: Cranberry juice

UK brand names: Cranberry juice is a food substance included only for its potential to interact with drug metabolism.

Average doses:

- There is no average amount – this is self-consumed

What form does it come in: Liquid and solid (fruit) form.

Does it interact with other medicines: Yes, the following interactions are known:

- Warfarin (anticoagulant) increases the actions.

MEDICINES OPTIMISATION IN PREGNANCY AND BREASTFEEDING

Some medicines are known to be harmful in pregnancy. They may affect the development of the baby or mean the baby is more likely to be born with a disability. Medicines may especially affect the baby during early development, i.e. within the first trimester (13 weeks). Thus, if medicines (prescribed or not prescribed) cannot be considered safe, avoidance is recommended. However, in pregnancy it may be necessary to continue treatments for long-term conditions and this is monitored with guidance provided. Questions may arise around different health conditions or treatments, for example in a teenage pregnancy the person may be taking medications for acne (e.g. Isotretinon (branded as Roaccutane), or Co-cyprindiol). Medicines optimisation here revolves around taking as little as possible and seeking alternatives when needed for issues such as the occasional headache or nausea. This can be challenging if multiple medications were taken beforehand but it is managed by the doctor and midwife according to need and guidance.

SUMMARY

Medicines are a valuable part of patient care and treatment. Medicines are chemicals and have the potential to be harmful as well as therapeutic. To be useful and therapeutic they need to be taken by patients in the right route, right time, right frequency and in the right way. This is complicated by multiple medicines, patients' beliefs or decisions to not take medicines or take more if their condition improves or deteriorates. Best practice is to ensure evidence-based prescribing and treatment with a focus on the best outcomes for patients or medicines optimisation. Nurses are key to ensuring this and this chapter has summarised the key issues and knowledge for developing their practice around this challenging area.

LEARNING FROM A CASE STUDY: TEST YOUR KNOWLEDGE

Arianna is a 59-year-old woman who has a history of back pain, asthma since childhood and depression for the last two years since losing her job and after a marriage break-up.

Her current medication is:

- lansoprazole (30 mg once daily)
- gabapentin (600 mg three times daily)
- tramadol (50 mg – 100 mg every 4-6 hours)
- salbutamol metered dose inhaler (2 puffs as required)
- beclomethasone (100 micrograms 2 puffs twice daily)
- mirtazapine (30 mg every night)
- zopiclone (7.5 mg every night)

She is due for review of her pain management. She has been suffering from pain and complaining of drowsiness yet insomnia and weight gain. She has also had low mood for the last two years and has tried multiple antidepressants. She cannot stop smoking and currently smokes 20 ciga-rettes a day. This presents a challenge to engage Arianna in self-care. She is ordering salbutamol for her asthma frequently on a monthly basis as it is not under control. Her pain does not seem to improve with her current pain medication and she says this makes her depression worse.

Most recent consultations have been for pain and management. Prior to that consultations were regarding low mood after the break-up of her marriage and poor sleep. Arianna is also complaining about increased breathlessness, and orders a salbutamol inhaler each month.

1   What are the issues for medicines optimisation?
2   Are there any safety risks here?
3   What makes you think Arianna is unclear about her symptoms management (e.g. breathing)?
4   What considerations are there for Arianna in relation to medicines optimisation?

IF I REMEMBER 5 THINGS FROM THIS CHAPTER:

1   Medicines are a component in the control or management of conditions or symptoms and frequently encountered by nurses.
2   Patient understanding, attitude or behaviours can impact optimal outcomes from medicines and cause problems or ineffective management or treatment.
3   Medicines optimisation is a key term to address the optimum use of medicines in part-nership with patients which may include stopping, starting or changing medicines or non-medication interventions such as lifestyle changes to improve patient outcomes.
4   Adverse effects can occur and will impact on medicine optimisation, and need to be reported.
5   Polypharmacy can make medicines use and adherence difficult as it can be confusing or cause other adverse effects, and is key to consider in patient interactions.

ANSWERS TO CASE STUDY QUESTIONS

1   Effects of the medicines, multiple medicines, adhering to the medicine regime (timing, dosing) and self-administration.
2   Drowsiness from the medicine effects, potential for falls, plus the potential problem with moving and self-care with uncontrolled asthma.
3   The number of inhalers used and the consequence of ineffective asthma control. Effective use of the inhaler and of the maximal dose needed. The counterproductive smoking of cigarettes whilst trying to control her asthma.
4   Review the role of the medicines and seek to work with Arianna. Polypharmacy may be an issue so support her understanding of her medicines and how to take them, her triggers and cycle of pain and low mood each making the other worse, adverse effects which worsen the symptoms, e.g. weight gain and insomnia. Address the issue of medicines adherence and outcomes in the short and long term. Potential considerations:

- Asthma – inhaler is ineffective – what about inhaler technique and timing.
- Drowsiness – due to breathing difficulties and inadequate rest. Compounded drowsiness from interaction of Zopiclone, Mirtazapine, Gabapentin and Tramadol.
- Pain – long-term lower back pain and use of Gabapentin needs review and whether appropriate since there are no neurological causes, and long-term side effects may include mood alterations.
- Low mood (depression) – not improved by medication so review and address alternatives or non-medication interventions.
- Weight gain – this is an adverse effect of Mirtazapine so if this is reviewed it may improve.

GO FURTHER

Age UK calls for a more considered approach to prescribing medicines for our older population: www.ageuk.org.uk/latest-press/articles/2019/august/age-uk-calls-for-a-more-considered-approach-to-prescribing-medicines-for-older-people/

Nearly 2 million older people on seven or more prescription medicines at risk of side effects that are severe in some cases, and occasionally even life threatening.

REFERENCES AND RECOMMENDED READING

de Jager, R.L., van Maarseveen, E.M., Bots, M.L. and Blankestijn, P.J. (2018) Medication adherence in patients with apparent resistant hypertension: Findings from the SYMPATHY trial. *British Journal of Clinical Pharmacology*, *84*(1): 18–24. doi:10.1111/bcp. 13402.

Insani, W.N., Whittlesea, C., Alwafi, H., Man, K.K.C., Chapman, S. and Wei, L. (2021) Prevalence of adverse drug reactions in the primary care setting: A systematic review and meta-analysis. *PLoS One*, *16*(5): e0252161. www.ncbi.nlm.nih.gov/pmc/articles/PMC8153435/

Joint Formulary Committee (2022) British National Formulary (online) London: BMJ and Pharmaceutical Press https://bnf.nice.org.uk/ (Accessed 20 February 2022)

Kaufman, G. (2015) Adverse drug reactions: Classification, susceptibility and reporting. *Nursing Standard*, *30*(50): 53–63. doi:10.7748/ns.2016.e10214.

The Kings Fund (n.d.) Long-term conditions and multi-morbidity. Available at: www.kingsfund.org.uk/projects/time-think-differently/trends-disease-and-disability-long-term-conditions-multi-morbidity

Medicines and Healthcare Regulatory Authority (2022) #FakeMeds campaign. Available at: https://fakemeds.campaign.gov.uk/

National Co-ordinating Centre for NHS Service Delivery and Organisation Research & Development (NCCSDO) (2005) Concordance, adherence and compliance in medicine taking. Available at: www.ahpo.net/assets/NCCSDO%20Compliance%202005.pdf

National Health England Medicines Optimisation (2015) Available at: https://www.england.nhs.uk/medicines-2/medicines-optimisation/

National Health Service Business Services Authority (NHSBA) (2022) Prescribing costs in hospitals and the community (2021–2022). Available at: www.nhsbsa.nhs.uk/statistical-collections/prescribing-costs-hospitals-and-community-england/prescribing-costs-hospitals-and-community-england-202122

National Institute for Health and Care Excellence (NICE) (2009) Medicines adherence: involving patients in decisions about prescribed medicines and supporting adherence. Lineal guideline [CG76]. Available at: www.nice.org.uk/guidance/cg76

National Institute for Health and Care Excellence (2015) Medicines optimisation: the safe and effective use of medicines to enable the best possible outcomes NICE guideline [NG5]. Available at: https://www.nice.org.uk/guidance/ng5; https://www.nice.org.uk/guidance/ng5/resources/medicines-optimisation-the-safe-and-effective-use-of-medicines-to-enable-the-best-possible-outcomes-pdf-51041805253

National Institute for Health and Care Excellence (NICE) (2016) Medicines optimisation. Quality standard [QS120]. Available at: www.nice.org.uk/guidance/qs120/chapter/quality-statement-4-medicines-reconciliation-in-acute-settings

National Institute for Health and Care Excellence (2024) Guidance. https://www.nice.org.uk/ (Accessed 20 February 2024)

Nieuwlaat, R., Wilczynski, N., Navarro, T., Hobson, N., Jeffery, R., Keepanasseril, A., Agoritsas, T., Mistry, N., Iorio, A., Jack, S., Sivaramalingam, B., Iserman, E., Mustafa, R.A., Jedraszewski, D., Cotoi, C. and Haynes, R.B. (2014) Interventions for enhancing medication adherence. *Cochrane Database of Systematic Reviews*. doi:10.1002/14651858.CD000011.pub4

Nursing and Midwifery Council (2018) Future nurse: Standards of proficiency for registered nurses. https://www.nmc.org.uk/globalassets/sitedocuments/standards-of-proficiency/nurses/future-nurse-proficiencies.pdf

Osanlou, R., Walker, L., Hughes, D.A. and Pirmohamed, M. (2022) Adverse drug reactions, multimorbidity and polypharmacy: A prospective analysis of 1 month of medical admissions. *BMJ Open, 12*: e055551. doi:10.1136/bmjopen-2021-055551.

Royal College of Nursing (RCN) and Royal Pharmaceutical Society (RPS) (2020) Guidance on prescribing, dispensing, supplying and administration of medicines. Available at: www.rpharms.com/Portals/0/RPS%20document%20library/Open%20access/Professional%20standards/SSHM%20and%20Admin/RCN%20RPS%20additional%20guidance.pdf?ver=2020-03-05-121229-987

Royal Pharmaceutical Society (RPS) (2013) Medicines optimisation: Helping patients to make the most of medicines. Available at: www.rpharms.com/Portals/0/RPS%20document%20library/Open%20access/Policy/helping-patients-make-the-most-of-their-medicines.pdf

Vrijens, B., De Geest, S., Hughes, D.A., Przemyslaw, K., Demonceau, J., Ruppar, T., Dobbels, F., Fargher, E., Morrison, V., Lewek, P., Matyjaszczyk, M., Mshelia, C., Clyne, W., Aronson, J.K. and Urquhart, J. (2012) ABC Project Team. A new taxonomy for describing and defining adherence to medications. *British Journal of Clinical Pharmacology, 73*(5): 691–705. doi:10.1111/j.1365-2125.2012.04167.x

World Health Organisation (WHO) (2017) *Medication Without Harm – Global Patient Safety Challenge on Medication Safety*. Geneva: World Health Organization. Licence: CC BY-NC-SA 3.0 IGO.

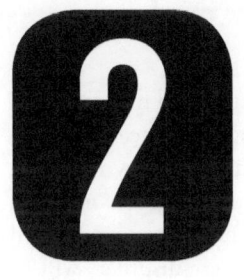

MEDICINES FOR INFLAMMATORY AND AUTOIMMUNE CONDITIONS

RACHAEL MAJOR

AFTER READING THIS CHAPTER YOU WILL BE ABLE TO:

- Outline the effect of the immune system has in the development of inflammatory and autoimmune disorders.
- Briefly discuss the actions of the drugs involved in treating inflammatory and autoimmune conditions.
- Discuss the drugs used to treat inflammatory and autoimmune conditions, considering the routes of administration and interactions.
- Apply knowledge of medicines to inform the holistic treatment of patients with inflammatory and autoimmune disorders.

OVERVIEW

The immune system plays a key role in defending the body from pathogens and foreign bodies which may cause harm to the individual. This system involves the complex interaction of many chemical mediators, proteins as well as white blood cells. The adaptive immune system recognises previously encountered antigens and will be able to mount a quicker and more robust response, however this can cause the individual difficulties if this is associated with unwanted or even dangerous symptoms such as anaphylaxis, allergic responses, asthma or eczema. In some individuals, the immune system does not recognise the individual's tissues as their own and therefore treats them as foreign, which causes autoimmune conditions such as rheumatoid arthritis, psoriasis, multiple sclerosis, systemic lupus erythematosus, myasthenia gravis and Grave's disease. Other immune conditions such as

Crohn's disease and ulcerative colitis may have a mixture of autoimmune and inflammatory causes. Medications for immune and autoimmune conditions often act to reduce the action of the immune system or act to reduce the effects caused by the inflammatory response. This chapter will review the drugs within these categories. While type 1 diabetes mellitus, thyroid disorders and Addison's disease are autoimmune disorders, they have a significant effect on the body's metabolism, and therefore drugs used to treat these disorders will be addressed in Chapter 4.

GO FURTHER

To refresh your knowledge on the immune system review your favourite physiology text-book or review the resources below:

- Simple video giving overview of the immune system: www.youtube.com/watch?v=1KdlU1sQcyc
- Autoimmune diseases: www.youtube.com/watch?v=2YK5vBUm9C8
- Hypersensitivity: www.youtube.com/watch?v=jXTW4F-8jd4

THE MEDICINES LIST

- Antihistamines
- Bronchodilators
- Leukotriene receptor antagonists
- Corticosteroids
- Xanthines
- Disease modifying antirheumatic drugs
- Immunosuppressants
- Non-steroidal anti-inflammatories (see Chapter 7).

DRUG GROUPS/CONCEPT: ANTIHISTAMINES

Antihistamines or H1-receptor antagonists that compete with histamine, which is released during an allergic reaction, for the H1 receptor sites. Antihistamines do not prevent the release of histamine but compete with histamine at the receptor sites and therefore will reduce the effect of histamine. Antihistamines are most effective if taken before histamine is released or when symptoms are first experienced (Willihnganz et al., 2020). Antihistamines are commonly categorised into sedating and non-sedating.

Drug group: Antihistamines – non-sedating

Drug name: Acrivastine

UK brand names: Benadryl Allergy Relief

Average doses:

- 8 mg three times a day

What form does it come in: Capsules

Does it interact with other medicines: Yes, the following interactions are known:

- May increase sedative effect of alcohol and central nervous system (CNS) depressants.
- Potential interaction with erythromycin, ketoconazole and grapefruit juice.

Drug name: Cetirizine hydrochloride

UK brand names: Benadryl Allergy, Zirtec Allergy, Allacan, Boots Hayfever and Allergy Relief, Piriteze Allergy, Pollenase Allergy and Hayfever Relief, POLLENSHEILD Hayfever Relief, Wockhardt Allergy and Hayfever Relief

Average doses:

- 10 mg once per day

What form does it come in: Tablets, liquid and capsules

Does it interact with other medicines: No

Drug name: Fexofenadine hydrochloride

UK brand names: Allevia, Almerg, Telfast, Treathay

Average doses:

- 120–180 mg per day

What form does it come in: Tablets

Does it interact with other medicines: Yes, the following interactions are known:

(Continued)

- The following decrease exposure to fexofenadine: apple and orange juice, apalutamide, lorlatinib, rifamycins.
- The following increase exposure to or concentration of fexofenadine: berotralstat, darolutamide, dronedarone, elexacaftor, eligustat, ibrutinib, ivacaftor, lapatinib, leflunomide, letermovir, mirabegron, neratinib, olaparib, osmimertinib, pibrentasvir, pitolisant, roxadustat, sotorasib, tepotinib, teriflunomide, tucatinib, vandetanib, velpatasvir, vemburafenib, venetoclaz.
- Aluminium and magnesium containing antacids reduce absorption.

Drug name: Loratadine

UK brand names: Boots Hayfever Relief, Boots One a Day Allergy Relief, Brown and Burk Once a Day Hayfever Relief, Clarityn Allergy

Average doses:

- 10 mg once daily

What form does it come in: Tablets and liquid

Does it interact with other medicines: Yes, the following interactions are known:

- Ketoconazole, erythromycin and cimetidine increase plasma concentrations of loratadine but without clinically significant changes.
- All known inhibitors of enzymes CYP3A4 or CYP2D6 result in elevated levels of loratadine which may increase side effects.

Drug group: Antihistamines – sedating

Drug name: Chlorphenamine maleate

UK brand names: Boots Allergy Relief, Piriton

Average doses:

- Orally 4 mg every 4-6 hours, maximum 24 mg per day for adults, maximum 12 mg per day for elderly
- By injection (intramuscular or intravenous): 10 mg, repeat if necessary up to four times a day

What form does it come in: Tablets, liquid, injection

Does it interact with other medicines: Yes, the following interactions are known:

- Chlorphenamine increases the risk of adverse effects with the following: clozapine, monoamine oxidase inhibitors, drugs causing sedation.

Drug name: Promethazine hydrochloride

UK brand names: Phenergan, Sominex

Average doses:

- Orally 10-20 mg, 2-3 times per day, or 25-50 mg for sedation or travel sickness
- By slow intravenous injection or deep intramuscular injection 25-50 mg

What form does it come in: Tablets and liquid

Does it interact with other medicines: Yes, the following interactions are known:

- Promethazine will increase the effects and potential adverse effects of: anticholinergics, tricyclic antidepressants, sedatives, hypnotics, alcohol, drugs known to cause prolongation of the QT interval in electrocardiographs (such as antiarrhythmics, antimicrobials, antidepressants and antipsychotics).

DRUG GROUPS/CONCEPT: BRONCHODILATORS

Beta 2 adrenergic agonists: these drugs act on beta 2 adrenergic receptors which are abundant in airway smooth muscle. Activation of these receptors triggers relaxation of airway smooth muscle through activation of intracellular second messengers. Beta 2 receptor agonists can be categorised into short acting (SABA) which have a half-life of 3–6 hours and long acting (LABA) which have a half-life of 18–24 hours or longer. Long-term use of beta 2 receptor agonists reduces their efficacy as this reduces the number of beta 2 receptors in airway smooth muscle. SABA are often used as rescue inhalers in acute asthma. Good inhaler technique is extremely important to ensure that the optimum dose of the drug is inhaled, and many patients benefit from the use of spacer devices to help with this. Potentially serious hypokalaemia can result from high use of beta 2 agonists and particular caution should be taken when administered with xanthines, corticosteroids and diuretics which will exacerbate this. Side effects of increased blood pressure, heart rate, tremors, feelings of palpitations and headache have all been reported.

Muscarinic receptor antagonists: Airway smooth muscle tone is mainly controlled by the parasympathetic nervous system and in particular by the neurotransmitter acetylcholine

(Cazzola et al., 2020). Muscarinic receptor antagonists act by blocking the action of acetylcholine and therefore reducing the contraction of smooth muscle. Muscarinic receptor antagonists are usually classified into short acting (SAMA) or long acting (LAMA) and can be combined with beta 2 adrenergic agonists and inhaled corticosteroids in the treatment of asthma and chronic obstructive pulmonary disease (COPD). The most common side effect noted is a dry mouth, although uncommon serious side effects associated with muscarinic antagonists include glaucoma, constipation and urinary retention; this is less common with inhaled preparations although risks increase with age.

GO FURTHER

Further guidance on the treatment of asthma can be found at:

- NICE guidelines for asthma: www.nice.org.uk/guidance/ng80/chapter/Recommendations #principles-of-pharmacological-treatment
- NICE guidelines for COPD: www.nice.org.uk/guidance/ng115

Drug group: Short-acting beta 2 adrenoreceptor agonists

Drug name: Salbutamol

UK brand names: Ventolin

Average doses:

- 2.5–5 mg four times per day by nebuliser or more frequently in severe cases
- 1-2 puffs up to four times a day or 2–10 puffs repeated every 10–20 minutes or when required for moderate to severe acute asthma

What form does it come in: Pressurised inhaler, nebuliser, liquid

Does it interact with other medicines: Yes, the following interactions are known:

- Non-selective beta adrenoreceptor agonists such as propranolol will reduce the effects.
- Xanthine derivatives, steroids or non-potassium sparing diuretics may potentiate risk of hypokalaemia.
- Atomoxetine, monoamine oxidase inhibitors and linezolid increase the risk of hypertension and adverse cardiovascular effects.

Drug name: Terbutaline sulphate

UK brand names: Bricanyl

Average doses:

- Inhalation – 500 micrograms up to four times a day; by mouth 2.5-5 mg three times a day; by injection 250-500 micrograms up to four times day; by continuous infusion 90-300 micrograms/hour for 8-10 hours; by nebuliser 5-10 mg, 2-4 times a day

What form does it come in: Tablets, inhalation powder, solution for injection, nebuliser liquid

Does it interact with other medicines: Yes, the following interactions are known:

- As salbutamol.

Drug group: Long-acting beta 2 adrenoreceptor agonists

Drug name: Olodaterol

UK brand names: Striverdi Respimat

Average doses:

- 2 puffs daily

What form does it come in: Inhalation solution

Does it interact with other medicines: Yes, the following interactions are known:

- Beta blockers.
- Xanthine derivatives, steroids or non-potassium sparing diuretics may potentiate risk of hypokalaemia.
- Atomoxetine, monoamine oxidase inhibitors and linezolid increase the risk of hypertension and adverse cardiovascular effects.

(Continued)

Drug name: Salmeterol

UK brand names: Serevent, Neovent, Soltel

Average doses:

- 50-100 micrograms twice daily

What form does it come in: Inhalation powder, pressurised inhaler

Does it interact with other medicines: Yes, the following interactions are known:

- Beta adrenoreceptor agonists.
- The following drugs increase the exposure to salmeterol: ketoconazole, cobicistat, idelalisib, HIV-protease inhibitors, macrolides, neurokinin-1 receptor antagonists.
- Monoamine oxidase inhibitors and linezolid increase the risk of hypertension and adverse cardiovascular effects.

Drug name: Formoterol

UK brand names: Atimos Modulite, Oxis Turbohaler, Foradil

Average doses:

- 6-12 micrograms 1-2 times daily

What form does it come in: Inhalation powder, pressurised inhaler

Does it interact with other medicines: Yes, the following interactions are known:

- As Olodaterol.

Drug name: Indacaterol

UK brand names: Onbrez Breezhaler

Average doses:

- 150-300 micrograms once daily

What form does it come in: Inhalation powder

Does it interact with other medicines: Yes, the following interactions are known:

- As Olodaterol.

Drug group: Short-acting muscarinic antagonists

Drug name: Ipratropium bromide

UK brand names: Atrovent, Ipravent

Average doses:

- 250–500 micrograms 3–4 times a day

What form does it come in: Nebuliser, pressurised inhaler

Does it interact with other medicines: Yes, the following interactions are known:

- Beta 2 agonists – may increase risk of acute glaucoma in patients with history of narrow angle glaucoma.

Drug group: Long-acting muscarinic antagonists

Drug name: Tiotropium

UK brand names: Spiriva, Braltus

Average doses:

- 1 inhaled capsule per day

What form does it come in: Nebuliser, pressurised inhaler

Does it interact with other medicines: No

Drug name: Glycopyrronium bromide

UK brand names: Seebri Breezhaler

Average doses:

- 1 inhaled capsule per day

What form does it come in: Inhaler (available in other forms to manage excess secretions)

Does it interact with other medicines: No

(Continued)

Drug name: Umeclidinium

UK brand names: Incruse Ellipta

Average doses:

- 1 inhaled dose per day

What form does it come in: Pressurised inhaler

Does it interact with other medicines: No

DRUG GROUPS/CONCEPT: CYSTEINYL LEUKOTRIENE RECEPTOR ANTAGONISTS

Cysteinyl leukotriene receptor antagonists act to block leukotriene receptors and therefore the action of leukotrienes at that site. Leukotrienes are inflammatory mediators which are released by the white blood cells, mainly eosinophils, mast cells, basophils and macrophages. These leukotrienes cause bronchospasm, vasodilation in blood vessel except coronary vessels, where vasoconstriction occurs, and contribute to anaphylaxis and asthma (Ritter et al., 2020)

Drug name: Montelukast

UK brand names: Singulair

Average doses:

- 10 mg daily

What form does it come in: Granules, chewable tablet, tablet

Does it interact with other medicines: No

DRUG GROUPS/CONCEPT: CORTICOSTEROIDS

Corticosteroids are one of the main drugs used for the treatment of inflammation across a wide range of conditions from asthma to inflammatory bowel disease. These drugs mimic the two types of corticosteroids in the body; glucocorticoids and mineralocorticoids. Mineralocorticoids act to regulate body sodium and water concentration and therefore affect blood pressure and will be addressed in more detail in Chapter 6; however, some of the drugs have mixed action and therefore this is worth noting. The glucocorticoids have many actions including metabolic actions of increasing blood glucose concentrations through gluconeogenesis and reducing cell uptake of glucose, breakdown of adipose tissue and increasing breakdown of proteins. Glucocorticoids also have anti-inflammatory and immunosuppressive effects, reducing the action and proliferation of inflammatory cells, inhibiting prostaglandin synthesis, reducing the production of immunoglobulins and reducing the release of inflammatory mediators such as cytokines (Ashelford et al., 2019).

Long-term steroid use can lead to Cushing's syndrome as well as other side effects such as adrenal suppression, immunosuppression, psychiatric reactions, osteoporosis, diabetes mellitus, osteoporosis, glaucoma and cataracts, peptic ulcers and skin thinning for topical preparations (Ashelford et al., 2019). A steroid treatment card is recommended for patients who are on high dose steroids for longer than three weeks and dosage must be reduced slowly to prevent potentially life-threatening adrenal crisis (NHS England, 2020). Local administration and using the lowest dose possible for the shortest time possible reduces the risks of side effects. Inhaled corticosteroids are indicated in the treatment of asthma and COPD (NICE, 2021).

Drug group: Inhaled corticosteroids

Drug name: Beclometasone

UK brand names: Clenil Modulite, Kelhale, Qvar, Soprobec

Average doses:

- 50–400 micrograms twice daily (depending on brand used)

What form does it come in: Inhalation powder, pressurised inhaler

Does it interact with other medicines: Yes, the following interactions are known (although risk low is for inhaled drugs):

- The following drugs may increase exposure to beclometasone: cobicistat, HIV-protease inhibitors, idealisib.

Drug name: Budesonide

UK brand names: Pulmicort, Easyhaler (budesonide), Budelin

Average doses:

- By inhalation: 200–400 micrograms once daily; by nebuliser: 0.25–2 mg twice daily

(Continued)

What form does it come in: Inhalation powder, nebuliser liquid

Does it interact with other medicines: Yes, the following interactions are known (although risk is low for inhaled drugs):

- CYP3A inhibitors, e.g. itraconazole, ketoconazole, HIV-protease inhibitors, cobicistat, may increase exposure.

Drug name: Fluticasone

UK brand names: Flixotide

Average doses:

- By inhalation: 100–500 micrograms twice daily; by nebuliser: 0.5–2 mg twice daily

What form does it come in: Inhalation powder, pressurised inhaler, nebuliser liquid

Does it interact with other medicines: Yes, the following interactions are known (although risk is low for inhaled drugs):

- CYP3A inhibitors, e.g. itraconazole, ritonavir, ketoconazole, HIV-protease inhibitors, cobicistat, may increase exposure.

Drug name: Mometasone furoate

UK brand names: Asmanex Twisthaler, Enerzair Breezhaler, Clarinaze Allergy Control Nasal, Nasonex Nasal Spray

Average doses:

- Initially 400 mg per day in 1-2 doses, then 200 mg daily for asthma. Nasal spray 50-200 mg daily for rhinitis

What form does it come in: Inhalation powder, spray

Does it interact with other medicines: Yes, the following interactions are known (although risk is low for inhaled drugs):

- CYP3A inhibitors, e.g. itraconazole, ritonavir, ketoconazole, HIV-protease inhibitors, cobicistat, may increase exposure.

Many of the drugs for asthma and COPD are found in combination in inhalers. These inhalers are shown it Table 2.1.

Table 2.1 Drug group: Combined inhalers

Name of inhaler	Short-acting beta agonist included	Long-acting beta agonist included	Short-acting muscarinic antagonist included	Long-acting muscarinic antagonist included	Corticosteroid included
Combivent, Ipramol	Salbutamol		Ipratropium bromide		
Spiolta Respimat		Olodaterol		Tiotropium	
Ulibro Breezhaler		Indacaterol		Glycopyrronium	
Fostair		Formoterol			Beclometasone
Trimbow		Formoterol		Glycopyrronium	Beclometasone
Symbicort, Duoresp Spiromax, Fobumix		Formoterol			Budesonide
Flutiform		Formoterol			Fluticasone
AirFluSal, Combisal, Fusacomb, Sereflo, Seretide		Salmeterol			Fluticasone
Atectura Breezhaler		Indacaterol			Mometasone furoate
Enerzair Breezhaler		Indacaterol		Glycopyrronium	Mometasone furoate

Drug group: Oral/ injectable corticosteroids

Drug name: Prednisolone

UK brand names: Prevanti, Pred Forte, Scheriproct

Average doses:

- Orally 10-100 mg daily, depending on treatment condition; rectally 5-20 mg 1-2 times a day

What form does it come in: Rectal foam, tablet, suppository, enema

Does it interact with other medicines: Yes, the following interactions are known:

(Continued)

- The following drugs increase the effects of prednisolone: oestrogens, ketoconazole, erythromycin, ritonavir, diltiazem.
- The following drugs decrease the effects of prednisolone: rifampicin, rifabutin, carbamazepine, phenobarbitone, phenytoin, primidone, adrenaline, aminoglutethimide, mifepristone, grapefruit juice.
- Potassium-reducing diuretics (thiazides, furosemide, ethacrynic acid) and other drugs that reduce potassium including amphotericin B, xanthines and beta 2 agonists – increased risk of hypokalaemia.
- Prednisolone increases the effects or side effects of the following drugs: atroprine and other anticholinergics, NSAIDs, methotrexate, CYP3A inhibitors including cobicistat, warfarin, fluoroquinolones, ciclosporin.
- Prednisolone decreases the effects of the following drugs: oral anticoagulants, anticholinesterases, hypoglycaemic agents (including insulin), anti-hypertensive, diuretics, isoniazid, somatotropin, tretinoin, vecuronium.

Drug name: Betamethasone

UK brand names: Betnesol

Average doses:

- 0.5-5 mg daily orally, 4-20 mg intramuscular, slow intravenous injection or intravenous infusion up to four times in 24 hours

What form does it come in: Soluble tablet, solution for injection

Does it interact with other medicines: Yes, the following interactions are known:

- As prednisolone.
- Betamethasone increases the metabolism of quetiapine.

Drug name: Deflazacort

UK brand names: Calcort

Average doses:

- Orally up to 120 mg initially, 3-18 mg daily maintenance dose

What form does it come in: Tablet

Does it interact with other medicines: Yes, the following interactions are known:

- As prednisolone.

Drug name: Dexamethasone

UK brand names: Glensoludex, Dexsol, Martapan, Neofordex

Average doses:

- Orally: 0.5-1 mg daily higher in palliative care and critical care; by intravenous injection: 4-16 mg daily depending on condition in palliative care

What form does it come in: Soluble tablet, tablet, solution for injection, liquid

Does it interact with other medicines: Yes, the following interactions are known:

- As prednisolone.

Drug name: Hydrocortisone

UK brand names: Plenadren, Hydventia, Solu-Cortef

Average doses:

- Orally 20-30 mg daily; by intravenous injection 50-100 mg every 6 hours or 100-300 mg depending on condition

What form does it come in: Tablet, soluble tablet, powder for injection, solution for injection

Does it interact with other medicines: Yes, the following interactions are known:

- As prednisolone.

Drug name: Methylprednisolone

UK brand names: Depo-medrone, Medrone, Solu-medrone

Average doses:

- Orally: 20-40 mg daily; by injection: 10 mg to 1 g daily, depending on condition being treated

What form does it come in: Powder for injection, tablets, suspension for injection

Does it interact with other medicines: Yes, the following interactions are known:

- As prednisolone.

Drug group: Topical corticosteroids

Drug name: Beclometasone dipropionate

UK brand names: None

Average doses:

- Apply 1-2 times daily, 250 micrograms per gram

What form does it come in: Cream, ointment

Does it interact with other medicines: No

Drug name: Betamethasone

UK brand names: Betnovate, Bettamousse, Betnovate-RD, Diprosone, Audivate, Betesil, Betacap

Average doses:

- Apply 1-2 times a day, 0.25-1 mg per gram

What form does it come in: Foam, medicated plasters, cream, ointment, liquid

Does it interact with other medicines: No

Drug name: Clobetasol

UK brand names: Clobaderm, Dermovate, Etrivex

Average doses:

- Apply 1-2 times daily for up to four weeks, 500 micrograms per gram

What form does it come in: Shampoo, cream, ointment, liquid

Does it interact with other medicines: No

Drug name: Fluticasone

UK brand names: Cutivate

Average doses:

- Apply 1-2 times daily 500 micrograms per gram

What form does it come in: Cream, ointment

Does it interact with other medicines: No

Drug name: Hydrocortisone

UK brand names: Dermacort, Mildison Lipocream

Average doses:

- Apply 1-2 times daily, 5-25 mg per gram

What form does it come in: Cream, ointment

Does it interact with other medicines: No

Drug name: Mometasone furoate

UK brand names: Elocon

Average doses:

- Apply once daily, 1 mg per gram

What form does it come in: Cream, ointment, liquid

Does it interact with other medicines: No

DRUG GROUP/CONCEPT: XANTHINES

Xanthines include Theophylline and Aminophylline. The precise mechanism of action of these drugs is unclear, however they relax airway smooth muscle, increase the contractility of the diaphragm, stimulate the respiratory system and have some anti-inflammatory properties (Pleasants, 2018).

Cautions

Theophylline (which is also the main constituent of aminophylline) has a narrow therapeutic index and therefore overdose can lead to potentially fatal toxicity. Signs of toxicity include tachycardia, nausea, vomiting, haematemesis, restlessness, agitation, hallucinations, extreme thirst, seizures, dilated pupils, palpitations, arrythmias, disturbed electrolyte balance including hypokalaemia, hyperglycaemia, respiratory and metabolic acidosis, and rhabdomyolysis can occur. Treatment includes the use of activated charcoal, antiemetics and reversal of electrolyte imbalances and diazepam or lorazepam for seizures and agitation.

Drug group: Xanthines

Drug name: Aminophylline

UK brand names: Phyllocontin Continuous, Phyllocontin Forte Continuous

Average doses:

- 250-500 mg by slow injection or 500-700 mg/kg/hour intravenous injection, 225-450 mg per day modified release tablets. Reduce dose for the elderly. Monitor blood theophylline levels.

What form does it come in: Solution for injection, modified release tablets

Does it interact with other medicines: Yes, the following interactions are known:

- The following drugs may increase plasma theophylline concentrations: fluvoxamine, cimetidine, macrolide antibiotics (e.g. erythromycin, clarithromycin), quinolone antibiotics (e.g. ciprofloxacin, norfloxacin), fluconazole, isoniazid, propranolol, allopurinol (high doses, e.g. 600 mg daily), oral contraceptives, mexiletine, propafenone, calcium channel blockers, (diltiazem, verapamil), Disulfiram, Interferon alfa, influenza vaccine, methotrexate, deferasirox, rucaparib, zafirlukast, tacrine, thiabendazole, thyroid hormones, valaciclovir, aciclovir.
- The following drugs may decrease plasma theophylline concentrations: rifampicin, antiepileptics (e.g. carbamazepine, phenytoin, primidone, phenobarbitone), ritonavir, leflunomide, aminoglutethiamide sulfinpyrazone, St John's wort, smoking, alcohol.
- Increased adverse effects have been noted when co-administered with the following drugs: quinolone antibiotics, cardiac glycosides, dosapram, halothane, ketamine, sympathomimetics, beta blockers, esketamine, lomustine.
- Aminophylline reduces the effects of the following drugs: beta adrenergic agonists, lithium, adenosine, zafirlukast, benzodiazepines, pancuronium.
- Hypokalaemia resulting from β2 agonist therapy, steroids, diuretics and hypoxia may be potentiated by xanthines.
- The effects of lithium are reduced.

Drug name: Theophylline

UK brand names: Uniphyllin Continuous

Average doses:

- 200–400 mg twice a day

What form does it come in: Modified release tablets. Monitor blood levels. Risk of severe side effects in the elderly

Does it interact with other medicines: Yes, the following interactions are known:

- As aminophylline.

DRUG GROUP/CONCEPT: DISEASE MODIFYING ANTI-RHEUMATIC DRUGS (DMARDS)

This is a wide group of drugs used to treat rheumatoid arthritis and, in some cases, inflammatory bowel disease and psoriasis, including methotrexate, sulfasalazine, penicillamine, gold complex (sodium aurothiomalate) and antimalarial drugs such as hydroxychloroquine, chloroquine and mepacrine (sometimes used in systemic lupus erythematosus). Methotrexate is a folic acid antagonist, but it has many actions that contribute to its anti-inflammatory effects including increasing adenosine release which suppresses many inflammatory and immune responses, increasing the sensitivity of T-cells to apoptosis and modulating cell-specific signalling pathways involved in inflammation (Cronstein and Aune, 2020).

Sulfasalazine acts by inhibiting the inflammatory cyclooxygenase and lipoxygenase pathways thus inhibiting the production of prostaglandins and leukotrienes, but also acts to reduce the release of interleukin-8 from colonic myofibroblasts (Ritter et al., 2020).

Drug name: Methotrexate

UK brand names: Maxtrex, Methofill, Metoject PEN, Nordimet, Zlatal

Average doses:

- 7.5–30 mg per week

(Continued)

What form does it come in: Tablet, intramuscular injection, intravenous injection, subcutaneous injection

Does it interact with other medicines: Yes, the following interactions are known:

- The following drugs increase the concentration of methotrexate: acetazolamide, nsaids, aspirin, acitretin, phenylbutazone, phenytoin, barbiturates, tranquilisers, oral contraceptives, darolutamide, levetiracetam, brigatinib, eltrombopag, leflunomide, nitisinone, metamizole, potassium aminobenzoate, para-aminobenzoic acid, protein pump inhibitors, regorafenib, thiazide diuretics, doxorubicin, tetracyclines, tedizolid, teriflunomide, probenecid, sulfinpyrazone, penicillin, glycopeptide antibiotic, trimethoprim, levetiracetam, sulfonamides, ciprofloxacin, cefalotin and oral hypoglycaemics.
- The following drugs decrease exposure to methotrexate: Acetazolamide, apalutamide.
- The following drugs affect the efficacy of methotrexate: asparaginase, crisantaspase, pegaspargase.
- The following drugs increase the risks of adverse reactions or toxicity when given with methotrexate: aminophylline, theophylline, aspirin (high dose), pyrimethamine, nitrous oxide, NSAIDs, penicillins, ciprofloxacin, tegafur, trimethoprim.
- Live vaccines can cause life-threatening infections.

Drug name: Hydroxychloroquine sulphate

UK brand names: Quinoric

Average doses:

- 220–400 mg per day

What form does it come in: Tablet

Does it interact with other medicines: Yes, the following interactions are known:

- The following drugs reduce the absorption or concentration of hydroxychloroquine: oral antacids, calcium salts, lanthanum.
- Hydroxychloroquine decreases the effects of the following drugs: agalsidase alfa and beta, rabies and cholera vaccines, laronidase, remdesivir, anti-epileptics.
- Hydroxychloroquine increases the effects of the following drugs: ciclosporin, hypoglycaemic drugs.
- Potential toxicity with penicillamine.
- Cimetidine increases the concentration of hydroxychloroquine.

Drug name: Leflunomide

UK brand names: Arava

Average doses:

- 100 mg initially for 3 days then 10–20 mg daily

What form does it come in: Tablet

Does it interact with other medicines: Yes, this drug interacts with many drugs including but not limited to:

- Leflunomide increases exposure to: agomelatine, anthracyclines, fexofenidine, furosemide, cephalosporins, bosentan, H2 receptor antagonists, methotrexate, NSAIDs, penicillins, pioglitazone, quinolone antibiotics, rifamycins, statins, sulfasalazine, sulfonylureas, taxanes.
- Leflunomide decreases exposure to: alpelisib, aminophylline, ropivacaine, clozapine olanzapine, baricitinib, caffeine, duloxetine, melatonin, theophylline.
- Increased risk of immunosuppression with: filgotinib.
- Leflunomide increases the effects of: coumarins (warfarin).
- Live vaccines can cause life-threatening infections.

Note this drug has a very long half-life and interactions may occur after it has been stopped.

Drug name: Penicillamine

UK brand names: None

Average doses:

- 125–750 mg daily

What form does it come in: Tablet

Does it interact with other medicines: Yes, the following interactions are known:

- The following drugs decrease the absorption of penicillamine: antacids, iron, zinc.
- The following drugs increase the risk of adverse reactions with penicillamine: chloroquine, hydroxychloroquine, gold.
- Penicillamine decreases the concentration of digoxin.

(Continued)

Drug name: Sulfasalazine

UK brand names: Salazopyrin

Average doses:

- For acute attack of ulcerative colitis or Crohn's disease 1-2 g four times a day orally or 0.5-1 g twice a day rectally in conjunction with oral therapy. Maintenance does 500 mg four times a day 0.5-1 g twice a day with or without oral therapy. For rheumatoid arthritis 500 mg daily increasing up to 2-3 g daily in divided doses

What form does it come in: Oral suspension, gastric resistant tablet, tablet, suppository

Does it interact with other medicines: Yes, the following interactions are known:

- The following drugs increase the exposure to sulfasalazine: antiandrogens, antifungals (azoles), leflunomide regorafenib tedizolid, teriflunomide, velpatasvir, ventoclax, voxilaprevir.
- Sulfasalazine decreases the concentration or absorption of: digoxin, folates.

DRUG GROUP/CONCEPT: IMMUNOSUPPRESSANTS

Immunosuppressant drugs are used to treat autoimmune conditions and to treat or prevent transplant rejection. Most of these drugs act to reduce lymphocyte proliferation during the inflammatory response but many also have additional actions. Ciclosporin and tacrolimus act to reduce the production of interleukin-2 (IL-2) which reduced the production of T cells (Ritter et al., 2020). Both drugs have the potential to be nephrotoxic and caution must be taken. Tacrolimus also increases blood potassium levels. Azathioprine interferes with purine synthesis (purines are found in both RNA and DNA) and is cytotoxic. It is widely used for immunosuppression and reduces both cell-mediated and antibody-mediated immune responses.

Biopharmaceuticals are engineered recombinant antibodies and other proteins including T-cell activation inhibitors, tissue necrosis factor (TNF) alpha inhibitors and interleukin inhibitors. These are expensive to produce, cannot be given orally and are generally limited to patients who have not responded to other DMARD therapy.

Janus kinase (JAK) inhibitors are the newest class of drugs used to treat rheumatoid arthritis and other inflammatory disorders. There are several different JAK subtypes, but these molecules interact with inflammatory cytokines and therefore inhibiting these molecules can reduce the inflammatory process (Harrington et al., 2020). JAK inhibitors include Baricitinib, Filgotinib, Tofacitinib and Upadacitinib.

As expected, treatment with immunosuppressants increases the risk of serious infection, especially in the elderly. Patients should continue to have routine vaccinations, although they are unable to have live vaccines such as BCG, shingles, varicella, yellow fever, oral typhoid, MMR, rotovirus and live influenza vaccine (children who are in close contact of immunosuppressed patients should receive inactivated influenza vaccine) (UK Health Security Agency, 2020).

Drug group: Immunosuppressants – antimetabolites

Drug name: Azathioprine

UK brand names: Azapress, Imuran

Average doses:

- 0.5–3 mg/kg daily

What form does it come in: Tablet, powder for injection

Does it interact with other medicines: Yes, the following interactions are known:

- The following drugs increase the risk of adverse reactions with azathioprine: ACE inhibitors, allopurinol, filgotinib.
- Azathioprine decreases the effects of coumarins (warfarin).
- Febuxostat increases exposure to azathioprine.

Drug group: Immunosuppressants – calcineurin inhibitors

Drug name: Ciclosporin

UK brand names: Sandimmun, Capsorin, Neoral, Capimune, Deximune, Vanquoral

Average doses:

- 1.5–2.5 mg/kg twice daily, higher in organ/bone marrow transplantation

What form does it come in: Capsule, solution for infusion, oral solution

Does it interact with other medicines: Yes, there are many interactions with this drug as it inhibits the metabolic enzyme CYP3A4 and transporter proteins involved in reducing drug availability. Examples of interaction include but are not limited to the following:

- The following drugs decrease ciclosporin levels: barbiturates, carbamazepine, oxcarbazepine, phenytoin, nafcillin, intravenous sulfadimidine, probucol, octreotide, orlistat, rifampicin, St John's Wort, ticlopidine, sulfinpyrazone, terbinafine, bosentan.
- All inhibitors of CYP3A4 and/or P-glycoprotein may lead to increased levels of ciclosporin. Examples are: amiodarone, azithromycin, antifungals (azoles), nicardipine, metoclopramide, oral contraceptives, methylprednisolone (high dose), allopurinol,

(Continued)

cholic acid and derivatives, protease inhibitors, imatinib, colchicine, nefazodone, diltiazem, verapamil, danazol, pomelo, purple grape and grapefruit juices.
- Ciclosporin increases levels of: anthracycline antibiotics, aliskiren, ambrisentan, digoxin, NSAIDs, colchicine, statins, repaglinide and etoposide.
- The following drugs increase the risk of nephrotoxicity when combined with ciclosporin: aminoglycosides (including gentamicin, tobramycin), amphotericin B, ciprofloxacin, vancomycin, trimethoprim (+sulfamethoxazole), bezafibrate, fenofibrate, NSAIDs, cimetidine, ranitidine, methotrexate, tacrolimus.

Drug name: Tacrolimus

UK brand names: Adoport, Advagraf, Dailiport, Envarsus, Modigraf, Prograf, Protopic

Average doses:

- By intravenous infusion: 10–100 micrograms/kg daily. By oral administration 75–300 micrograms/kg per day

What form does it come in: Modified release tablet, granules, modified release capsule, solution for infusion

Does it interact with other medicines: Yes – there are many interactions with this drug as it is metabolised by CYP34A and also inhibits this enzyme. Examples of interaction include but are not limited to the following:

- The following drugs increase blood levels of tacrolimus: antifungals (azoles), macrolide antibiotics, ritonavir, nelfinavir, saquinavir, telaprevir, boceprevir, ritonavir, letermovir, cobicistat, nilotinib, imatinib, clotrimazole, clarithromycin, josamycin, nifedipine, nicardipine, diltiazem, verapamil, amiodarone, danazol, ethinylestradiol, omeprazole, nefazodone, lansoprazole and ciclosporin, metoclopramide, cimetidine and magnesium-aluminium-hydroxide, NSAIDs, oral anticoagulants, or oral antidiabetics, cannabidiol, bromocriptine, cortisone, dapsone, ergotamine, gestodene, lidocaine, mephenytoin, miconazole, midazolam, nilvadipine, norethisterone, quinidine, tamoxifen, troleandomycin, pomelo, pomegranate and grapefruit juices.
- The following drugs reduce blood levels of tacrolimus: rifampicin, phenytoin, St John's Wort, phenobarbital, corticosteroids, carbamazepine, metamizole, isoniazid, metamizole, flucloxacillin.
- Tacrolimus increases levels of: ciclosporin, phenytoin, oral contraceptives, pentobarbital, phenazone, mycophenolic acid.
- The following drugs increase the risk of nephrotoxicity when combined with: aminoglycosides, gyrase inhibitors, vancomycin, sulfamethoxazole with trimethoprim, NSAIDs, ganciclovir, aciclovir, amphotericin B.
- Potassium sparing diuretics increase the risk of hyperkalaemia.

Drug group: Immunosuppressants – JAK inhibitors

Drug name: Baricitinib

UK brand names: Olumiant

Average doses:

- 4 mg daily

What form does it come in: Tablet

Does it interact with other medicines: Yes, the following interactions are known:

- Filgotinib increases risk of immunosuppression.
- Leflunomide and teriflunomide increase levels of baricitinib.

Drug name: Filgotinib

UK brand names: Jyseleca

Average doses:

- 200 mg daily

What form does it come in: Tablet

Does it interact with other medicines: Yes, the following interactions are known:

- Increased risk of immunosuppression with: abatacept anakinra azathioprine, baricitinib, ciclosporin, etanercept, leflunomide, monoclonal antibodies, tacrolimus, teriflunomide.
- Tofacitinib increases the risk of immunosuppression.
- Filgotinib increases the levels of the following drugs: angiotensin II receptor antagonists (valsartan), fexofenadine, endothelial receptor antagonists, glibenclamide, repaglinide, statins.

Drug name: Tofacitinib

UK brand names: Xeljanz

Average doses:

- 5 mg daily

(Continued)

What form does it come in: Tablet

Does it interact with other medicines: Yes, there are many interactions with this drug including but not limited to the following:

- The following drugs decrease levels of tofacitinib: antiandrogens, dronedarone, antiepileptics, mitotane, NNRTIs, rifamycins, St John's Wort.
- The following drugs increase levels of tofacitinib: antifungals (azoles), diltiazem, verapamil, ciclosporin, cobicistat, crizotinib, HIV-protease inhibitors, macrolides (clarithromycin, erythromycin) neurokinin 1 receptor antagonists, SSRIs (selective serotonin reuptake inhibitors, such as fluoxetine, fluvoxamine), nilotinib, tacrolimus.
- Filgotinib increases the risk of immunosuppression.

Drug name: Upadacitinib

UK brand names: Rinvoq

Average doses:

- 15 mg daily

What form does it come in: Tablet

Does it interact with other medicines: Yes, the following interactions are known:

- The following drugs decrease levels of upadacitinib: antiandrogens, antiepileptics, mitotane, rifamycins.
- The following drugs increase levels of upadacitinib: antifungals (azoles), cobicistat, HIV-protease inhibitors, idelalisib, macrolides (clarithromycin).

Drug group: Immunosuppressants – interleukin inhibitors

Drug name: Sarilumab

UK brand names: Kezara

Average doses:

- 200 mg every two weeks

What form does it come in: Solution for injection

Does it interact with other medicines: Yes, the following interactions are known:

- Sarilumab reduces levels of the following drugs: aminophylline, ciclosporin, combined hormonal contraceptives, coumarins (warfarin), sirolimus, statins, tacrolimus, theophylline.
- Filgotinib increases the risk of immunosuppression.

Drug name: Tocilizumab

UK brand names: RoActemra

Average doses: 162 mg weekly by subcutaneous injection or 8 mg/kg every four weeks by intravenous infusion

What form does it come in: Solution for injection, solution for infusion

Does it interact with other medicines: Yes, the following interactions are known:

- Tocilizumab reduces levels of the following drugs: aminophylline, antiepileptics, benzodiazepines, calcium channel blockers, ciclosporin, corticosteroids, coumarins (warfarin), statins, theophylline.
- Filgotinib increases the risk of immunosuppression.

Drug group: Immunosuppressants - T cell activation inhibitors

Drug name: Abatacept

UK brand names: Orencia

Average doses:

- 500 mg - 1 g every 2-4 weeks by infusion, or 125 mg weekly by subcutaneous injection

What form does it come in: Powder for infusion, solution for injection

Does it interact with other medicines: Yes, the following interactions are known:

- Filgotinib and monoclonal antibodies increases the risk of immunosuppression and severe infection.

Drug group: Immunosuppressants – tumour necrosis factor alpha (TNFα) inhibitors

Drug name: Adalimumab

UK brand names: Amgevita, Humira, Hyrimoz, Idacio, Imraldi, Yuflyma

Average doses:

- Initial 160 mg dose for Crohn's disease (accelerated pathway), ulcerative colitis and hidradenitis suppurativa; 80 mg initially for Crohn's disease, plaque psoriasis and uveitis. Then 40 mg every two weeks by subcutaneous injection

What form does it come in: Solution for injection

Does it interact with other medicines: Yes, the following interactions are known:

- Filgotinib increases the risk of immunosuppression.

Drug name: Certolizumab pegol

UK brand names: Cimzia

Average doses:

- 400 mg every two weeks for 3 doses then 200 mg every two weeks

What form does it come in: Solution for injection

Does it interact with other medicines: Yes, the following interactions are known:

- As adalimumab.

Drug name: Etanercept

UK brand names: Benpali, Enbrel

Average doses:

- 25 mg twice weekly or 50 mg weekly

What form does it come in: Solution for injection, powder, solvent for injection

Does it interact with other medicines: Yes, the following interactions are known:

- As adalimumab.

Drug name: Golimumab

UK brand names: Simponi

Average doses:

- For ulcerative colitis 200 mg initially then 100 mg after two weeks, then 50-100 mg every four weeks. For rheumatoid arthritis, ankylosing spondylitis, non-radiographic axial spondylitis and psoriatic arthritis 50-100 mg once a month

What form does it come in: Solution for injection

Does it interact with other medicines: Yes, the following interactions are known:

- Anakinra and filgotinib increases the risk of immunosuppression.

Drug name: Infliximab

UK brand names: Flixabi, Inflectra, Remicade, Remsima, Zessly

Average doses:

- Initially 5 mg/kg by intravenous infusion then 5 mg/kg after two weeks then a further 5 mg/kg six weeks after initial dose. Maintenance dose 5 mg/kg every eight weeks. If taken with methotrexate initial doses are 3 mg/kg increasing to a maximum of 7.5 mg/kg every eight weeks. Maintenance dose by subcutaneous injection 120 mg every two weeks)

What form does it come in: Solution for injection, powder for infusion

Does it interact with other medicines: Yes, the following interactions are known:

- As adalimumab.

DRUG GROUP/CONCEPT: NON-STEROIDAL ANTI-INFLAMMATORIES (NSAIDS)

NSAIDs are covered further in Chapter 7.

GO FURTHER

Further information on drugs used in rheumatoid arthritis can be found on the National Rheumatoid Arthritis Society website: https://nras.org.uk/resource/medicines-in-rheumatoid-arthritis/

MEDICINES FOR INFLAMMATORY AND AUTOIMMUNE CONDITIONS IN PREGNANCY AND BREASTFEEDING

With pregnancy and breastfeeding the risks and benefits to the pregnant person and baby or foetus need to be balanced. Medication for asthma and COPD, including oral corticosteroids if absolutely required, should be continued to maintain good control.

Many autoimmune disorders are less active during pregnancy and therefore patients may experience fewer symptoms. It is important, if possible, to stabilise the person before any planned pregnancy on drugs that are safe to use. These include NSAIDs, ciclosporin, corticosteroids, sulfasalazine and hydroxychloroquine at the lowest effective dose. Methotrexate and leflunomide should be stopped. Methotrexate is known to cause miscarriage and foetal abnormalities. Leflunomide metabolites persist for a long time and a washout procedure may be required in the case of unplanned pregnancy to reduce the risk to the foetus. Monoclonal antibodies readily cross the placenta, so in general manufacturers advise against pregnancy whilst on this treatment and for six months after the last dose. If pregnancy does occur, limited studies have shown an increase in infection in pre-term babies, and infants must not have live vaccines for six months (Pham-Huy et al., 2021). Manufacturers of JAK inhibitors advise avoiding use in pregnancy as foetal toxicity has been seen in animal studies.

Most manufacturers advise against the use of antihistamines during pregnancy although there is no evidence that they cause foetal abnormalities. There is some evidence that use in the third trimester can cause irritability and tremor in the newborn (Joint Formulary Committee, 2024) and that antihistamines are present in breast milk.

GO FURTHER

UK teratology information service: https://uktis.org/monographs/

LEARNING FROM A CASE STUDY: TEST YOUR KNOWLEDGE

Jalissa is a 19-year-old student who has been brought into the emergency department following an acute asthma attack. They were initially treated with a salbutamol nebuliser driven by oxygen on admission and their breathing has improved but they still have an audible wheeze. On questioning Jalissa can answer in short bursts of a couple of words and states that they had been prescribed two different inhalers. They show you a salbutamol inhaler which is empty. They cannot name the other inhaler but although they were told to take it daily, they have not done so for several weeks as they did not feel they needed it. They stated that they had just moved into student accommodation which was damp and had not been feeling well with a cold for several days.

1   What second inhaler might Jalissa have been prescribed?
2   Why do certain types of inhalers need to be taken regularly?
3   Why was Jalissa prescribed salbutamol via a nebuliser?
4   What health promotion and follow-up might Jalissa require in relation to their medication for asthma?

IF I REMEMBER 5 THINGS FROM THIS CHAPTER:

1   Many of the drugs in this chapter are used to treat a wide variety of inflammatory and autoimmune disorders by regulating aspects of the immune system.
2   Many of the inflammatory conditions are chronic and painful. They have a huge impact on the patient's life. Medication aims to reduce the symptoms and increase quality of life.
3   Many patients will have tried a number of drugs in this chapter to get an optimum response.
4   Polypharmacy and drug interactions have to be considered. Many of these drugs will be initiated by specialist practitioner.
5   A holistic approach is required to maintain medicine optimisation and quality of life.

ANSWERS TO CASE STUDY QUESTIONS

1   Jalissa is likely to have been prescribed an inhaled corticosteroid as per NICE guidelines (https://cks.nice.org.uk/topics/asthma/management/newly-diagnosed-asthma), along with the short-acting beta agonist salbutamol if they were using the salbutamol regularly, or if they had symptoms three times a week or were being woken up with asthma symptoms once a week.
2   Preventer inhalers, such as inhaled corticosteroids or those with long-acting beta agonists, are designed to reduce the likelihood of asthma attacks by reducing inflammation and by causing longer-term bronchodilation. It can take 1-3 weeks for inhaled corticosteroids to have a maximum effect although they can start working in 24 hours and should be taken even if asthma is well controlled.
3   Nebulisers, especially if driven by oxygen, reduce hypoxia and push the medication into the lungs. They do not rely on inhaler technique which can be especially poor during an acute asthma attack when the patient is tiring and therefore a higher drug concentration can be delivered to where it is needed.
4   Jalissa will need advice on when to take their inhalers and inhaler technique. They will need follow-up review to check on progress. Their home situation may also be exacerbating their asthma.

REFERENCES AND RECOMMENDED READING

Ashelford, S., Raynsford, J. and Taylor, V. (2019) *Pathophysiology and Pharmacology in Nursing* (2nd edn). London: Sage Publishing.

Calija, B. (2017) Microsized and Nanosized Carriers for Nonsteroidal Anti-Inflammatory Drugs Formulation Challenges and Potential Benefits. London: Elsevier.

Cazzola, M., Rogliani, P. and Matera, M.G. (2020) The latest on the role of LAMAs in asthma. *Journal of allergy and clinical immunology*, *146*(6): 1288–1291.

Cronstein, B.N. and Aune, T.M. (2020) Methotrexate and its mechanisms of action in inflammatory arthritis. *Nature Reviews Rheumatology*, *16*: 145–154. https://doi.org/10.1038/s41584-020-0373-9

Datapharm (2023) Electronic medicines compendium. Available at: www.medicines.org.uk/emc

Harrington, R., Al Nokhatha, S.A. and Conway, R. (2020) JAK inhibitors in rheumatoid arthritis: An evidence-based review on the emerging clinical data. *Journal of Inflammation Research*, *30*: 519–531.

Joint Formulary Committee (2024) British National Formulary. Available at: https://bnf.nice.org.uk/ (Accessed: 21 February 2024).

National Institute for Health and Care Excellence (NICE) (2023) Inflammatory bowel disease. Available at: www.nice.org.uk/guidance/conditions-and-diseases/digestive-tract-conditions/inflammatory-bowel-disease

National Institute for Health and Care Excellence (NICE) (2021) Asthma: Diagnosis, monitoring and chronic asthma management. NICE guideline [NG80]. Available at: www.nice.org.uk/guidance/ng80

National Institute for Health and Care Excellence (NICE) (2020) Rheumatoid arthritis in adults: Management. NICE guideline [NG100]. Available at: www.nice.org.uk/guidance/ng100

National Institute for Health and Care Excellence (NICE) (2017) Psoriasis: Assessment and management. Available at: www.nice.org.uk/guidance/cg153/chapter/1-Recommendations#systemic-therapy

NHS England (2020) Steroid Emergency Card to support early recognition and treatment of adrenal crisis in adults. Available at: https://www.england.nhs.uk/2020/08/steroid-emergency-card-to-support-early-recognition-and-treatment-of-adrenal-crisis-in-adults/

Pham-Huy, A., Top, K.A., Constantinescu, C., Seow, C.H. and El-Chaâr, D. (2021) The use and impact of monoclonal antibody biologics during pregnancy. *Canadian Medical Association Journal*, *193*(29): E1129–E1136. doi:10.1503/cmaj.202391.

Pleasants, R. (2018) Clinicial pharmacology of oral maintenance therapies for obstructive lung diseases. *Respiratory Care*, *63*(6): 671–689.

Ritter, J.M., Flower, R., Henderson, H., Kong Loke, Y., MacEwan, D. and Rang, H.P. (2020) *Rang and Dale's Pharmacology* (9th edn). Edinburgh: Elsevier.

UK Health Security Agency (2020) The green book. Available at: www.gov.uk/government/collections/immunisation-against-infectious-disease-the-green-book#the-green-book

Willihnganz, M.J., Gurevitz, S.L. and Clayton, B.D. (2020) *Clayton's Basic Pharmacology for Nurses*. St Louis: Elsevier.

3 MEDICINES FOR INFECTIONS

SHEILA CUNNINGHAM

AFTER READING THIS CHAPTER YOU WILL BE ABLE TO:

- Describe what is meant by infection and the principles of treatment.
- Explain and differentiate between antiviral, antifungal and antibiotic drugs.
- Outline the key consideration and issues with the use of antimicrobial drugs.
- Consider and reflect on how you would apply knowledge around antimicrobial drug treatments to support clinical decision making.

WHEN DO WE NEED MEDICINES FOR INFECTIONS?

There are huge numbers of microorganisms which people come into contact with every day either within food, the environment or even within healthcare settings. These microorganisms can be too small to see and may be beneficial or harmful (Richards and Edwards, 2020). In every clinical area where one finds patients there are approaches to keep people safe and avoid infections. However, infections do occur and this needs management through drug and non-drug means. These drugs are referred to as 'antimicrobials' which can also sometimes be referred to as 'chemotherapy' agents. These drugs are designed to treat infections by being 'selectively toxic' to invading infectious microorganisms whilst having minimal effects on the human (host) (Ritter et al, 2024). This group of drugs is broad including antibiotics, antivirals, antifungals and antiparasitics and the naming convention refers to the specific organisms intended for elimination. Success in developing drugs to eliminate invaders as above has faced equal and opposite microorganism success in developing means to resist the drugs.

HOW DO INFECTIONS OCCUR?

Bacteria are found in most areas including on and within humans. Most bacteria are harmless or considered helpful (termed commensals) such as those located in the bowel (e.g. *Escherichia coli* required for vitamin absorption and food breakdown), but some are pathogens or disease causing. This is for a number of reasons including located in a non-hospitable location, i.e. from one person to another, or from a benign area like the skin to a vulnerable and destructive area like a wound. Infections by pathogens, either viral, bacterial or others can cause significant health problems or even death for patients. Control of the spread of infection is imperative and nurses are very familiar with the 'cycle of infection' and skills to break this to prevent transmission of microorganisms and infections (Cunningham, 2017). Nonetheless, if organisms do invade and cause an infection this can be treated, such as bacterial infections being treated with antibiotics, which broadly work to either eliminate the organism (bactericidal) or impede its growth (bacteriostatic). Terminology varies and the collective term 'antimicrobials' is often used, but specifically within reference sources such the British National Formulary (JFC, 2022) these are expanded to specific groups of medicines: antibiotics (bacteria), antivirals (viruses), antifungals (fungi) and antiparasitics (parasites and worms).

Antibiotics are antimicrobials which impede the growth of bacteria. Antibiotics are commonly classified based on their mechanism of action, chemical structure or spectrum of activity. More specifically, narrow spectrum antibiotics target specific types of bacteria, such as Gram-negative or Gram-positive bacteria, whereas broad spectrum antibiotics affect a wide range of bacteria. Bacteriostatic antibiotics include the groups tetracyclines, macrolides, clindamycin, trimethoprim/sulfamethoxazole, linezolid and chloramphenicol (the routine clinical use of chloramphenicol has reduced in recent years because of its side effects). Since the action of bacteriostatic antimicrobials is to inhibit growth of bacteria, they require a functioning host (human) immune system to fully eliminate the remaining bacterial growth. Bactericidal (or bacteria-killing) antibiotics include the drug groups beta-lactams (i.e. penicillins, cephalosporins), daptomycin, fluoroquinolones, metronidazole, nitrofurantoin, co-trimoxazole and vancomycin. They impede bacteria by stopping the bacteria from making proteins, which is essential for survival and multiplication. Others interfere with their ability to copy DNA. Penicillin, the first antibiotic to be developed as a medicine, blocks the construction of the bacterial cell wall and thus impedes its integrity and it then ruptures. Daptomycin disrupts the integrity of the cell membrane, allowing ions or small molecules to leak in and out of the cell, which can also be lethal to bacteria (eMC, 2021: Summary of Product Characteristics).

Some antibacterials have been associated with a range of adverse effects. Side effects range from mild (rash, nausea) to very serious (anaphylaxis) depending on the antibiotics used, the microbial organisms targeted and the individual patient response. Some antibacterials impede normal bacterial growth (commensals), for example *Escherichia coli* which regulates physiological activity, leading to effects such as diarrhoea.

Viruses

Viral diseases such as measles, influenza and Covid-19 and many others result from viruses. These are small entities consisting of a protein coat (nucleocapsid) and a core of ribonucleic acid (RNA) or deoxyribonucleic acid (DNA) collectively referred to as a virion. Viruses cause infection by entering cells through connection to a surface protein receptor and entering by endocytosis and then altering cell functioning. They do not survive independently outside of a cell like bacteria do but rely on the cell nutrients and composition to aid their replication and multiplication, eventually bursting out of the cell to invade adjacent cells. Depending on their composition (DNA or RNA) the nucleus and DNA or

RNA of the host cell becomes the source of materials for the virus to manufacture copies of itself. Once inside a host cell the host immune system cannot see a virus until cells employ complex processes of 'presenting' segments of virus on the surface in specific proteins (called MHC) which informs the immune surveillance system (T cells) that viruses are inside. T cells then release cytotoxic chemical to kill the infected cell and, therefore, prevent the survival of the invading virus. These processes and chemicals contribute to the symptoms expressed by the infected person. Since viruses 'hijack' many of the metabolic processes of host cells it is a challenge to find drugs specific to viruses. Most antiviral agents are only effective when the virus is dividing (reproducing, also called replicating) and these agents which are generally enzymes target the differing stages of this to impede growth and thus prevent the virus from causing harm.

Fungi

Fungi can be single celled or very complex multicellular organisms. They are found in just about any habitat but most live on the land, mainly in soil or on plant material rather than in sea or fresh water. Whilst many are parasitic or saprophytic (ie living off dead matter) most fungi live harmlessly in the environment, contributing to food sources (mushrooms), manufacturing (yeast and brewing or production of antibiotics) or the carbon cycle through decay processes (Royal Botanic Gardens Kew 2020), Ritter et al, 2024). Some fungi however are pathogenic. Fungal infections are not usually serious in well and healthy adults. Often these can be referred to in relation to the parts of the body affected as superficial, subcutaneous or systemic, of which the latter is the more serious. Examples include *Candida albicans* (commonly known as 'thrush') or *Tinea pedis* (athlete's foot), which whilst uncomfortable or unsightly are not serious. Infections such as these can spread through 'auto-inoculation' or one infected part of the body infecting another. As athletes foot can spread to the groin, so guidance on clothing and hygiene accompanies drug therapy. However, patients who are vulnerable or immunocompromised are at risk of serious fungal infections, especially if they have had multiple courses of antibiotics (removing inbuilt protection from local bacteria) or been exposed to invasive procedures. Some fungi, for example yeasts, are simple structures and exist as single cells (Gould, 2011). Some complex forms exhibit branching structures (hyphae) which become a knitted mesh or 'mycelium' reminiscent of a moss structure on stones. Yeasts themselves produce spores which are hardy and may be spread via dust or on surfaces. Fungal infections are termed 'mycotic' and in the main in fit individuals are superficial, such as nail onychomycosis or those on skin or mucous membranes. The fungal infections caused by *Aspergillus* and *Candida* may become systemic and prove fatal especially in immunocompromised patients.

Issues

It is recognised that since the advent of powerful antimicrobial drugs, bacteria, viruses, fungi and parasites have adapted in response to them and increasingly no longer respond the same way. This makes infections harder to treat and increases the risk of disease spread, severe illness and death. The issue of drug resistance then is an important one in the prescription and use of these drugs, and the term 'antimicrobial stewardship' was coined to address this for practitioners (NICE, 2015; WHO, 2021). The emergence and spread of drug-resistant pathogens that have acquired new resistance mechanisms, leading to anti-microbial resistance, continues to threaten our ability to treat common infections. It is of concern that the multi-resistant (to many antibiotics) and pan-resistant (to all antibiotics) bacteria – commonly referred to in the media as 'superbugs' – are not treatable with existing antimicrobial medicines such as antibiotics, and they have and continue to spread globally (WHO, 2021).

Common bacterial infections, such as urinary tract infections, sepsis, sexually transmitted infections and some forms of diarrhoea are frequently treated with a core group of antibiotics. Prescribing is one issue here, but others include patient practice in taking antimicrobials, i.e. missing doses, sharing with others or ceasing if feeling better, contributing to non-completion of courses of antimicrobials. All this has contributed to antimicrobial resistance, resulting in less effective antibiotics.

Antimicrobial resistance is a global issue as it impacts on control of common infections, which is a leading concern in global public health. Since nurses are at the forefront of patient and client care it is a key responsibility in caring for patients safely to be antibiotic 'competent' (RCN, 2023). Antibiotic shortages and very slow antimicrobial innovation and develop-ment are affecting countries of all levels of development, especially in health care systems. In 2019 WHO identified 32 antibiotics in clinical development that address the WHO list of priority pathogens for which new antibiotics are needed based on their level of danger/ risk for control: for example *Pseudomonas aeruginosa*, which is multi-resistant, or methicillin-resistant *Staphylococcus aureus* or MRSA. The WHO also advise that the search for and develop-ment of new antibiotics is incredibly costly. The cost of antimicrobial resistance to national economies and their health systems is significant as it affects the productivity of patients or their caretakers through prolonged hospital stays and the need for more expensive and intensive care.

Some antibiotics have a very low therapeutic index and need careful monitoring when being administered. That means there is a narrow range between toxic and effective blood levels of the drug. These drugs are invariably administered in hospital or monitored situa-tions for that reason, as toxicity may be severe and irreversible. Examples of these drugs are gentamicin, aminoglycosides and vancomycin.

Individuals may also exhibit allergic responses to certain antibiotics, notably penicillin or cephalosporins, and care is needed if they do have an allergy as anaphylaxis is potentially life threatening. In most cases, the allergic reaction is mild to moderate and can take the form of: a raised, itchy skin rash (urticaria, or hives) and coughing. Common side effects not considered as penicillin 'allergy' also occur, which are uncomfortable but not life threatening and include:

- Delayed onset diarrhoea and vomiting
- Nausea
- Bloating and indigestion
- Abdominal pain
- Loss of appetite

GO FURTHER

Read this guidance for more information: Royal College of Nursing and Cardiff University (n.d.) Antimicrobial competency in stewardship. Available at: www.cardiff.ac.uk/_data/assets/pdf_file/0009/1391913/Updated-AMS-Competencies-7th-December-2020-updated-04.02.21.pdf

---

You now ought to have a good understanding of what causes infectious diseases, the different antimicrobials available for treatment and why antimicrobial stewardship is so important. Now there will be an opportunity to look at particular medicines in more detail, covering some of the main antibiotics, antifungal and antiviral drugs will be addressed in their own sections.

THE MEDICINES LIST

There are hundreds of different types of antibiotics, but most of them can be classified into six groups:

- Penicillins – these are widely used to treat a variety of infections, including skin infections, chest infections and urinary tract infections.
- Cephalosporins – these are used to treat a wide range of infections, but some are also effective for treating more serious infections, such as septicaemia and meningitis.
- Aminoglycosides – these tend to only be used in hospital to treat very serious illnesses such as septicaemia, as they can cause serious side effects. They are generally given by injection, but may be given as drops for some ear or eye infections.
- Tetracyclines – are broad-spectrum antibiotics and can be used to treat a wide range of infections, but whose value has decreased owing to increasing bacterial resistance.
- Macrolides – can be particularly useful for treating lung and chest infections. They possess an antibacterial spectrum that is similar but not identical to that of penicillin so is an alternative for people with a penicillin allergy, or to treat penicillin-resistant strains of bacteria.
- Fluoroquinolones – are broad-spectrum antibiotics that were once used to treat a wide range of infections, especially respiratory and urinary tract infections. These antibiotics are no longer used routinely because of the risk of serious side effects.
- Other – some antibacterials are semisynthetic or synthetics and include: chloramphenicol (eye and ear infections), fusidic acid (skin and eye infections) and trimethoprim (urinary tract infections).
- Anti-fungal drugs:
  o polyenes
  o imidazoles
- Antivirals:
  o viral DNA polymerase inhibitors
  o anti-replication

ANTIBACTERIAL DRUGS

Drug group: Penicillins

Drug name: Phenoxymethylpenicillin

UK brand names: Penicillin VK

Average doses:

- Adults: 250-500 mg every 6 hours (reduce for elderly with renal failure)
- Children 1-5 years: 125 mg every 6 hours; 6-12 years: 250 mg every 6 hours

What form does it come in: Film-coated tablets

Duration of therapy: 5-10 days (depending on infection)

Instructions: Each tablet should be swallowed whole with water, at least 30 minutes before food, as ingestion of phenoxymethylpenicillin with meals slightly reduces the absorption of the drug.

Does it interact with other medicines: Yes, the following interactions are known:

- Uricosuric drugs, e.g. probenecid and sulfinpyrazone - increases excretion of uric acid in urine.
- Warfarin and some other anticoagulants - may prolong prothrombin time.

Drug group: Cephalosporins

Drug name: Cefalexin

UK brand names: Cefadroxil, Cefazolin, Cefradine

Average doses:

- Adults: 250 mg every 6 hours, alternatively 500 mg every 8-12 hours; increased to 1-1.5 g every 6-8 hours, increased dose to be used for severe infections

What form does it come in: Capsules, tables and suspensions

Duration of therapy: 5-10 days (depending on infection)

Does it interact with other medicines: Yes, the following interactions are known:

- Colistimethate (particularly intravenous) which is a powerful antibiotic active against Gram-negative organisms including *Pseudomonas aeruginosa* and *Klebsiella pneumoniae*. Potentially increases the risk of nephrotoxicity when given with cefalexin.

Drug group: Tetracycline

Drug name: Tetracycline

UK brand names: Demeclocycline hydrochloride, Doxycycline, Lymecycline and Minocycline

Average doses:

- Adults: 250-500 mg every 6 hours (reduce for elderly with renal failure)

What form does it come in: Film-coated tablets

Duration of therapy: 7-10 days (depending on infection may be longer)

Instructions: Each tablet should be swallowed whole with water, at least 30 minutes before food, as ingestion of phenoxymethylpenicillin with meals slightly reduces the absorption of the drug. Tetracycline should be given one hour before or two hours after meals, since food and some dairy products interfere with absorption. The tablets should be taken with plenty of water. Therapy should be continued for up to three days after symptoms have subsided.

Does it interact with other medicines: Yes, the following interactions are known:

- Aenocoumarol, warfarin, phenindionel: increase anticoagulant effect by tetracycline. Manufacturer advises monitoring clotting (prothrombin time).
- Isotretinoin: acne medication increases the risk of serious benign intracranial hypertension when given with tetracycline – best to avoid concurrent use.
- Lithium: increased risk of lithium toxicity – it is recommended to avoid this.

Drug group: Macrolides

Drug name: Erythromycin

UK brand names: Azithromycin, Clarithromycin

Average doses:

- Adults: 250-500 mg 6 hourly increased to 500-1000 mg 6 hourly if the infection is very severe.

What form does it come in: Film-coated tablets or injectable solution

Duration of therapy: 5-7 days (depending on infection)

(Continued)

Cautions: Risk of cardiotoxicity (QT interval prolongation) so avoid in patients with cardiac disease or heart failure, conduction disturbances (MHRA advice, December 2020).

Does it interact with other medicines: Yes, hepatotoxicity and effects on the hepatic enzymes cytochrome P450 cause elevation or reduction in other drugs. Some examples are:

- Erythromycin causes increased serum concentrations of: acenocoumarol, alfentanil, astemizole, bromocriptine, carbamazepine, cilostazol, cyclosporin, digoxin, dihydroergotamine, disopyramide, ergotamine, hexobarbitone, methylprednisolone, midazolam, omeprazole, phenytoin, quinidine, rifabutin, sildenafil, tacrolimus, terfenadine, domperidone, theophylline, triazolam, valproate, vinblastine and antifungals, e.g. fluconazole, ketoconazole and itraconazole.
- Rifampicin, phenytoin, carbamazepine, phenobarbital and St John's Wort induce cytochrome P450 enzymes and may induce the metabolism of erythromycin, reducing serum concentrations.

Drug group: Fluoroquinolones

Drug name: Ciprofloxacin

UK brand names: Ciprox, Delafloxacin, Levofloxacin, Moxifloxacin, Ofloxacin

Average doses:

- Adults: 500–750 mg twice daily (alteration in dose for patients with renal and hepatic impairment)
- Children: 10–120 mg/kg (maximum dose 750 mg) depending on severity of infection

What form does it come in: Film-coated tablets, eye drops/ointment, intravenous solution

Duration of therapy: Three days (urinary tract infections or cystitis), 7–14 days (respiratory tract infections, skin infections)

Instructions: Oral tables should not be chewed; can be taken independent of meals but not with dairy products or mineral-fortified fruit juice.

Does it interact with other medicines: Yes, there are several theoretical interactions, some considered potentially serious; a few of these are:

- Aceclofenac, celecoxib, bromfenac, diclofenac (analgesia) potentially increases the risk of seizures.
- Ibuprofen, indomethacin, naproxin (potentially increases the risk of seizures).
- Clozapine (increased level of clozapine).
- Methotrexate (toxicity).

Drug group: Other (not in category above)

Drug name: Trimethoprim

UK brand names: Trimethoprim

Average doses:

- Adults: 200 mg twice a day for 7 days (up to 14 days if symptoms persist)
- Children over 12 years: Same as adult dose
- Children 6–12 years: 100 mg twice daily
- Children under 6: not suitable

What form does it come in: Tablets or oral suspension

Duration of therapy: 3–7 days (up to 14 days if symptoms persist)

Instructions: None specific – complete the course prescribed.

Does it interact with other medicines: Yes, the following interactions are known:

- Anticoagulants, e.g. acenocoumarol and warfarin – potentially increases anticoagulant effect.
- Colistimethate (antibiotics) increases risk of neptrotoxicity.
- Phenytoin and digoxin potentially increases the effects of these.

(Continued)

Drug name: Chloramphenicol

UK brand names: Eykappo, Minims

Average doses:

- Adults: Eye drops – one drop every 2 hours; eye ointment – at night. Ear drops – 2-3 drops, 2-3 times a day; oral capsules (in severe infections only in supervised situations) 500 mg (2 capsules) every 6 hours or 50 mg per kg body weight daily in divided doses
- Children: Eye drops – one drop every 2 hours; eye ointment – at night. Ear drops – 2-3 drops, 2-3 times a day. Oral capsules are not suitable (safety not established)

What form does it come in: Capsule, powder for solution for injection, solution preparations (ear drops, eye drops), eye ointment

Duration of therapy: Ear or eye solution: 5 days. Oral capsules under medical advice (severe infections)

Instructions: Eye drops/ointment: contact lenses should not be worn during the course of treatment. Ear drops: after instilling drops patients are advised to lie down with the affected ear uppermost for a minimum of 10 minutes.

Caution: Chloramphenicol oral capsules should only be used if other treatments are ineffective and its use should always be carefully monitored.

Does it interact with other medicines: Eye and ear preparations are not absorbed systemically so no interactions but caution is advised if hypersensitivity appears. The following interactions are known:

- Glibenclamide, tolbutamide and glicizide (antidiabetic medication of the sulfonylurea group) – risk of increased levels of these drugs.
- Phenytoin – increases levels.
- Tacrolimus (immunosuppressive drug) – increases levels.

Drug group: Fusidic acid

Drug name: Fusidic acid

UK brand names: Fucidin

Average doses:

- Adults: Cream/ointment: small amount topically to cover affected area 3-4 times a day. Eye ointment: twice a day. Oral: 500 mg every 8 hours

- Children: Cream/ointment: small amount topically to cover affected area 3-4 times a day. Eye ointment twice a day
- Children 12-17 years only: Oral: 500 mg every 8 hours

What form does it come in: Tablet, oral suspension, modified-release drops, powder and solvent for solution for infusion, topical cream and ointment

Duration of therapy: Cream/ointment for maximum one to two weeks. Oral for one week.

Instructions: None specific.

Caution: Oral tablets: not to be taken with statins or signs of hypersensitivity; extreme caution in people with liver or biliary disease.

Does it interact with other medicines: Yes, the following interactions are known with oral preparations:

- Atorvastatin, fluvastatin (and other statins) - increased risk of a condition called rhabdomyolysis (destruction of muscle tissue).

ANTIFUNGAL DRUGS

There are a range of antifungal preparations for either oral, genital skin or systemic fungal infections. The latter is considered extremely serious and hence these drugs are administered in a hospital setting. Several of these drugs have proprietary names and are well known to patients and the public, however they do have the same precautions and information needs as any drug.

Drug group: Polyenes

Drug name: Nystatin

UK brand names: None

Average doses:

- Adults and children: Oral suspension 1 ml (100,000 units) four times a day; cream/ointment (5 mg or 100,000 IU/g) apply sparingly to affected area. Weekly dose should not exceed 50 g/week

What form does it come in: Oral suspension, creams

Duration of therapy: Oral suspension and cream/ointment: 7 days

(Continued)

Instructions: None specific

Does it interact with other medicines: No

Drug name: Amphoteracin

UK brand names: Abelcet, Ambizone, Fungizone

Average doses:

- Adults: Abelcet: Test dose 1 mg, to be given over 15 minutes, then 5 mg/kg once daily for at least 14 days. Ambizone: Test dose 1 mg, to be given over 10 minutes, then 3 mg/kg once daily; maximum 5 mg/kg per day. Fungizone: Test dose 1 mg, to be given over 20-30 minutes, then 250 micrograms/kg daily, gradually increased over 2-4 days, increased if tolerated to 1 mg/kg daily, max (for severe infection)

What form does it come in: Suspension of intravenous infusion, powder injectable route

Duration of therapy: maximum 14 days for Ambicet, 7 days for Ambizone and Fungizone

Instructions: Intravenous use only often via an infusion pump in a hospital setting under qualified practitioner supervision.

Cautions: Only for very severe systemic fungal infections. Very toxic

Does it interact with other medicines: Yes, the following interactions are known:

- The following are implicated as causing severe hypokalaemia or nephrotoxicity:
  - Cancer treatments such as: apalutamide, bosutinib, cabozantinib, carboplatin (and others)
  - Bedaquiline (for tuberculosis)
  - Dexamethosone
  - Diclofenac
  - Disopyramide
  - Digoxin
  - Droperidol
  - Encorafenib
  - Erythromycin
  - Escitalopram
  - Other antifungals: fluconazole, flucytosine

- o   Antibiotics: gentamicin
- o   Antivirals: ganciclovir
- o   Haloperidol
- o   Hydroxychloroquine
- o   Hydroxyzine
- o   And many others (see BNF interactions: amphotericin).

Drug group: Imidazoles

Drug name: Clotrimazole

UK brand names: Canestan

Average doses:

- Adults: Topical (skin) use: thin layer of cream or spray over affected area 2-3 times a day
- Intravaginal (10% preparation) 5 g once only
- Intravaginal pessaries: 200 mg for 3 nights or one 500 mg pessary for one night

What form does it come in: Pessary, liquid, cream, spray

Duration of therapy: 1-5 days depending on formulation

Caution: Cream and pessaries may damage latex condoms and diaphragms.

Does it interact with other medicines: No

ANTIVIRAL DRUGS

As mentioned most antiviral drugs are enzymes by action to impede viral reproduction and proliferation. Development of newer drugs aims to impede viruses in other ways, e.g. from entering cells or impeding viral assembly. Antiviral drugs are categorised either in reference to the viral replication stage in which they work or according to the clinical conditions. It is recommended for some viruses which occur regularly such as the influenza virus, due to their ability to mutate and evolve, that illness is better prevented through vaccination. However, this section will address antiviral drugs rather than vaccination.

Drug group: Viral DNA polymerase inhibitor

Drug name: Aciclovir

UK brand names: Zovirax

Average doses:

- Adults: Tablets or oral suspension: 200 mg to 400 mg (depending on condition) 4 hourly (five times a day)
- For varicella zoster – chickenpox or herpes zoster – shingles: 800 mg, five times a day
- Creams: 1 g of cream containing 50 mg aciclovir. Thin film of cream should be applied to the infected and immediately adjacent skin areas 5 times daily

What form does it come in: Tablets, dispersible tablet, oral suspension, solution for infusion, eye ointment, cream

Duration of therapy: Tablets (for herpes simplex): 5 days; varicella or herpes zoster: 10 days

Does it interact with other medicines: Yes, the following interactions are known:

- Aminophylline, theophylline – increases level.
- Colistimethate – risk of nephrotoxicity.

Drug group: Anti-replication (influenza A and B)

Drug name: Oseltamivir

UK brand names: Tamiflu

Average doses:

- Adults weighing 24–40 kg: 60 mg twice daily
- Adults weighing over 41 kg: 75 mg twice daily

What form does it come in: Capsule, oral suspension, oral solution

Duration of therapy: 5 days

Instructions: The use of antivirals for the treatment and prevention of influenza should be determined on the basis of official recommendations. It is not a substitute for vaccination.

Does it interact with other medicines: No

Drug name: Zanamivir

UK brand names: Relenza

Average doses:

- Adults: Prophylaxis: 10 mg inhaled once a day
- Adults: Treatment: 10 mg inhaled twice a day

What form does it come in: Inhalation powder, solution for infusion

Duration of therapy: Prophylaxis – 10–28 days; treatment – 5 days

Instructions: Caution is needed with inhalation powder if the patient has asthma

Does it interact with other medicines: No

ANTIBIOTICS IN PREGNANCY AND BREASTFEEDING

Antibiotics can be generally tolerated during pregnancy. Some antibiotics do cross through breast milk and can be passed on to the baby, however these are often in very small amounts. Examples of antibiotics which may be considered safe include: amoxycillin, azithromycin, cefaclor, cefuroxime, cephalexin, clarithromycin co-amoxiclav and augmentin. However, there are a few antibiotics known to be 'teratogenic', that is they affect the growing foetus and should be avoided entirely during pregnancy (NHS, 2019; UKTIS, 2022). These include streptomycin and kanamycin (which may cause hearing loss) and tetracycline (which can lead to weakening, hypoplasia and discolouration of long bones and teeth) full details of these can be found in the British National Formulary or on the Summary of Product Characteristics sheet which accompanies all medicines.

CONSIDERATIONS WITH ANTIMICROBIALS

Effective antimicrobials are required for preventing and curing infections which could protect patients from potentially fatal diseases. For the many infections which are self-limiting (i.e. they will resolve on their own) antimicrobials (antibiotics) are not appropriate; however if prescribed then patients need to be supported to understand that they do need to take the entire course of medication until finished. Patient should not store antibiotics for use another time as this contributes to antimicrobial resistance and poor control of infections. Similarly, patients may request antibiotics for sore throats or colds but since these are viral infections antibiotics will do very little. The role of the nurse, alongside ensuring patients are supported and informed on how to take their medicines, is to be mindful of antibiotic stewardship in reducing antibiotic waste and resistance.

SUMMARY

This chapter addressed key aspects of infectious diseases and the approaches to managing them with medicines. There is a key responsibility to be 'frugal' with antibiotics in particular as so many microorganisms are becoming resistant to them. This does not obviate the need for knowledge of infection control, but adds the need for care planning and skills to manage and control infections appropriately.

LEARNING FROM A CASE STUDY: TEST YOUR KNOWLEDGE

Jenna (29 years old) arrives at the emergency department with dyspnoea, muscle pain (myalgia) and copious nasal secretions (rhinorrhoea). The symptoms began approximately two days ago and she reports feeling steadily worse. Jenna is having significant nasal secretions but minimal coughing. Her 4-year-old son has had rhinorrhoea as well over the past three days, but is not as ill as she is. She has had no other conditions and takes no routine medications. She was a smoker but gave up when she became pregnant. She is asking for antibiotics as she feels she has 'flu' and is worried as she needs to take care of her son. She tested for Covid but is negative.

1   What information (objective and subjective) might you collect from Jenna?
2   Reviewing how influenza affects body cells and tissues how might you discuss the illness with Jenna?
3   What are Jenna's medicine options? Are antibiotics justified?

IF I REMEMBER 5 THINGS FROM THIS CHAPTER:

1   Infectious diseases are caused by microorganisms; the main examples causing common diseases are bacteria, viruses and fungi.
2   Antimicrobial drugs include antibiotics, antivirals, antifungals as well as other antimicrobial classes, e.g. antiprotozoan. All work to inhibit the growth of or kill these infectious organisms.
3   Antimicrobials are specific to the organism, thus antibiotics which inhibit or eliminate bacteria will have no effect on viruses.
4   Drug formulations for antimicrobials are vast, indicating a range of routes and means to interfere with the microbes, for example topical preparations, inhalational, tablets for systemic use. All these work on the organism at the site of infections if localised and restricted.
5   Antimicrobials have been subject to misuse, excessive prescribing and if needed the full course ought to be completed to eliminate the organisms and not allow residual resistant organisms to survive, which can be more dangerous in the longer term.

ANSWERS TO CASE STUDY QUESTIONS

1   Subjective information: what is the colour of her nasal and bronchial secretions, does she have a fever, is she smoking again, does she have asthma, is she breathless and when. Objective information: temperature, pulse and blood pressure. Observe if her throat is red and sore, maybe take a swab. Ask if she usually has influenza vaccines, and if so has she had one.

2   You could explain this is a viral illness (seasonal cold) and contagious but self-limiting. The body is fighting the virus and as such there are signs and symptoms like feeling hot, maybe a fever, coughing and nasal secretions to act as a barrier and block further damage to cells and tissues. The main effects are due to the immune system working, not the virus.

3   Jenna's medicines ought to be symptomatic: an analgesic such as paracetamol for headaches, muscle aches and any fever. Wearing suitable clothing, ventilation and generally hot drinks and rest; if needed decongestants as in cold preparations but not with concurrent paracetamol due to the risk of taking an excess dose. Antibiotics are designed to combat bacteria – colds are viruses and thus the antibiotics would not work.

REFERENCES AND RECOMMENDED READING

Cunningham, S. (2017) Infection control. In T. Moore and S. Cunningham (eds), *Clinical Skills for Nursing Practice*. pp. 439–471. London: Routledge.

Electronic Medicines Compendium (eMC) (2021) daptomycin. Available at: www.medicines.org.uk/emc/product/177/smpc#PHARMACOLOGICAL_PROPS

Gould D. (2011) Diagnosis, prevention and treatment of fungal infections. *Nursing Standard*, 25(33):38-47; quiz 48. doi: 10.7748/ns2011.04.25.33.38.c8464.

Joint Formulary Committee (2022) British National Formulary (online) London: BMJ and Pharmaceutical Press. https://bnf.nice.org.uk/ (Accessed 20 February 2024)

National Health Service (NHS) (2019) Medicines in pregnancy. Available at: www.nhs.uk/pregnancy/keeping-well/medicines/

National Institute for Health and Care Excellence (NICE) (2015) Antimicrobial stewardship: Systems and processes for effective antimicrobial medicine use. NICE guideline [NG15]. Available at: www.nice.org.uk/guidance/ng15

Medicines and Healthcare Regulatory Authority (2020) Erythromycin: caution required due to cardiac risks (QT interval prolongation); drug interaction with rivaroxaban. Available at: https://www.gov.uk/drug-safety-update/erythromycin-caution-required-due-to-cardiac-risks-qt-interval-prolongation-drug-interaction-with-rivaroxaban

Public Health England (PHE) (2015) Guidance: Health matters: antimicrobial resistance. Available at: www.gov.uk/government/publications/health-matters-antimicrobial-resistance/health-matters-antimicrobial-resistance

Richards, A. and Edwards, S. (2020) *A Nurse's Survival Guide to Drugs in Practice*. London: Elsevier.

Ritter, J.M., Flower, R.J., Henderson, G., Loke, Y.K., MacEwan, D., Robinson, E. and Fullerton, J. (2024) *Rang & Dale's pharmacology* (10th edn). Elsevier Health Sciences.

Royal Botanic Gardens Kew (2020) Secret fungi in everyday life. Available at: https://www.
kew.org/read-and-watch/everyday-fungi-food-medicine

Royal College of Nursing (RCN) (2023) Antimicrobial resistance. Available at: www.rcn.org.
uk/clinical-topics/Infection-prevention-and-control-advice/Antimicrobial-resistance

UK Tetralogy Information Service (UKTIS) (2022) BUMPS – best use of medicines in pregnancy.
Available at: https://uktis.org/information-leaflets-for-pregnant-women/

World Health Organisation (WHO) (2021) Antimicrobial resistance. Available at: www.who.
int/news-room/fact-sheets/detail/antimicrobial-resistance

4 MEDICINES FOR METABOLIC CONDITIONS

RACHAEL MAJOR

AFTER READING THIS CHAPTER YOU WILL BE ABLE TO:

- Recognise the difference between the treatment of type 1 and type 2 diabetes mellitus.
- Discuss the pharmaceutical treatment of diabetes mellitus, thyroid disorders, Cushing's syndrome/disease and Addison's disease.
- Apply knowledge around medicines for metabolic conditions to support clinical decision making.

OVERVIEW

Metabolism is a set of reactions within the body and within cells that provide the body with energy to sustain life. This chapter will consider medications that are used to control conditions that affect metabolism.

The main metabolic disorder is diabetes mellitus with nearly 4 million affected in the UK in 2018–2019, 90% of those with type 2 (Diabetes UK 2020). Type 1 diabetes is an autoimmune disorder where the beta cells of the islets of Langerhans in the pancreas are not producing insulin. In type 2 diabetes adipose, skeletal muscle and liver cells become resistant to insulin and insufficient insulin is produced by the pancreas, causing raised blood glucose.

Insulin is required for glucose to enter cells to be used in cellular metabolism, as well as enhancing the synthesis of glycogen and therefore the storage of excess glucose. Insulin also increases the storage of fat, lipogenesis and lipid uptake into adipose cells. Insulin also stimulates the transport of free fatty acids to the liver and inhibits the catabolism of proteins (Seifter et al., 2022). Uncontrolled hyperglycaemia can have long-term effects such as retinopathy, nephropathy and neuropathy as well as increased risk of infections and vasculitis and increased atherosclerosis and therefore cardiovascular and renal disease. Hyperglycaemia can also lead to diabetic ketoacidosis or hyperosmotic hyperglycaemic nonketotic syndrome, both of which can cause death. Type 1 diabetes has to be treated with insulin, however patients with type 2 diabetes may still produce insulin and therefore treatments initially focus on diet and lifestyle, followed by drugs that reduce glucose absorption or excretion, increase insulin secretion or increase the sensitivity of cells to insulin.

Thyroid hormones are responsible for maintaining the metabolic rate, increasing adenosine triphosphate synthesis and consumption as well as heat production. They also promote normal growth and development in the foetus and in childhood (Seifter et al., 2022). Abnormally high levels of thyroid hormones can be caused by thyroid nodules, a pituitary tumour, high iodine intake or too high a dose of thyroid hormones, although the most common cause is Graves' disease, an autoimmune disorder. Hypothyroidism is most commonly an autoimmune disorder where thyroid cells are destroyed, but also can be the result of treatment for hyperthyroidism.

The glucocorticoids play a crucial role in the body's response to stress, the regulation of protein, glucose and fat metabolism and inflammation. Cushing's disease can be caused by exogenous or endogenous glucocorticoids leading to symptoms of fat redistribution, hyperglycaemia, hypertension, osteoporosis, muscle weakness, skin thinning, depression and hirsutism in women.

Addison's disease or primary adrenal insufficiency is where the body is not producing enough of the hormones produced by the adrenal cortex, in particular aldosterone and cortisol. This is usually an autoimmune disorder. Stress can cause a potentially life-threatening condition called Addisonian crisis and replacement therapy is urgently required.

This chapter will review the most common medications for the treatment of type 1 and type 2 diabetes mellitus as well as thyroid disorders, Cushing's disease and Addison's disease. The drugs will be presented in their drug groups below.

GO FURTHER

To learn more about these conditions please go to the following sites:

- Type 1 and Type 2 diabetes: www.youtube.com/watch?v=XfyGv-xwjll www.diabetes.org.uk/professionals
- Thyroid disorders: www.youtube.com/watch?v=S1kdYd4JGbg
- Cushing's syndrome: www.youtube.com/watch?v=v-jUwEpIzkE
- Addison's disease: www.youtube.com/watch?v=V6XcBp8EV7Q

THE MEDICINES LIST

- Insulins
- Blood glucose lowering drugs:
  - Alpha glucosidase inhibitors
  - Biguanides
  - Dipetidylpeptidase-4 inhibitors (gliptins)
  - Glucagon-like peptide-1 receptor agonists
  - Meglitinides

- ○ Selective glucose co-transporter 2 inhibitors
- ○ Thiazolidinediones (glitazones)
- Anti-thyroid drugs
- Thyroid hormones
- Drugs to treat Cushing's disease
- Drugs to treat Addison's disease

DRUG GROUPS/CONCEPT: INSULINS

Insulin is an anabolic hormone which facilitates the uptake and storage of glucose, amino acids and fats after a meal, reducing blood glucose. Normally insulin is released in two phases, a rapid initial release followed by a second phase which is slower and more prolonged until glucose levels are low enough not to trigger insulin release. Insulins are used primarily in type 1 diabetes to replace the deficiency, although it may also be required in type 2 diabetes as the disease progresses. Insulins used therapeutically have been developed to provide different onsets and durations of action. Soluble insulin produces a rapid and short-lived action; analogue insulins have been developed to be absorbed more quickly than plain insulin. Longer-acting insulins have been manipulated to slow the release of insulin from subcutaneous tissue. Diabetic control is often maintained by a combination of different types of insulin, although rapid acting insulins are used in insulin pumps. Porcine insulins are extracted from pig pancreases and are more likely to elicit an adverse immune response than recombinant insulins.

GO FURTHER

To learn more about the typical insulin profiles including duration of action please follow this link: www.diabetes.org.uk/resources-s3/2017-10/University%2520Hospitals%2520 of%2520Leicester%2520-%2520Insulin%2520Profiles.pdf

Drug group: Insulins – rapid-acting

Drug name: Insulin (insulin injection; neutral insulin; soluble insulin – short acting)

UK brand names: Actrapid, Humulin R, Humulin S, Hypurin Porcine Neurtal, Insuman Infusat, Insuman Rapid

Average doses:

- By subcutaneous or intramuscular injection, intravenous injection or infusion according to requirements

(Continued)

What form does it come in: Solution for injection

Does it interact with other medicines: Yes, the following interactions are known:

- Other antidiabetic drugs increase risk of hypoglycaemia.
- Fibrates increase risk of hypoglycaemia.

Drug name: Insulin aspart (recombinant human insulin analogue - short acting)

UK brand names: Fiasp, Novorapid

Average doses:

- By subcutaneous injection immediately before meals or shortly after meals when necessary. By subcutaneous or intravenous infusion according to requirements. Note that dosages of Fiasp and Novorapid are not interchangeable as Fiasp has a quicker onset of action and shorter duration

What form does it come in: Solution for injection including insulin pen refills

Does it interact with other medicines: Yes, the following interactions are known:

- As insulin.

Drug name: Insulin glulisine (recombinant human insulin analogue - short acting)

UK brand names: Apidra, Apridra soloStar

Average doses:

- By subcutaneous injection immediately before meals or shortly after meals when necessary. By subcutaneous or intravenous infusion according to requirements.

What form does it come in: Solution for injection

Does it interact with other medicines: Yes, the following interactions are known:

- As insulin.

Drug name: Insulin lispro (recombinant human insulin analogue - short acting)

UK brand names: Humalog, Lyumjev

Average doses:

- By subcutaneous injection immediately before meals or shortly after meals when necessary. By subcutaneous or intravenous infusion according to requirements.

What form does it come in: Solution for injection including insulin pen refills

Does it interact with other medicines: Yes, the following interactions are known:

- As insulin.

Drug group: Insulins - intermediate acting

Drug name: Biphasic isophane insulin

UK brand names: Humulin M3, Hypurin Porcine 30/70, Insuman Comb

Average doses:

- By subcutaneous injection according to requirements

What form does it come in: Suspension for injection

Does it interact with other medicines: Yes, the following interactions are known:

- As insulin.

Drug name: Isophane insulin; isophane protamine insulin injection; isophane insulin (NPH) - intermediate acting

UK brand names: Humulin I, Hypurin Porcine Isophane, Insulatard, Insulatard Innolet, Insuman Basal

Average doses:

- By subcutaneous injection: administer up to 15 minutes before food or shortly after according to requirements

(Continued)

What form does it come in: Suspension for injection

Does it interact with other medicines: Yes, the following interactions are known:

- As insulin.

Drug group: Insulins – intermediate acting combined with rapid acting

Drug name: Biphasic insulin aspart

UK brand names: Novomix 30

Average doses:

- By subcutaneous injection – administer 10 minutes before or shortly after a meal according to requirements

What form does it come in: Suspension for injection

Does it interact with other medicines: Yes, the following interactions are known:

- As insulin.

Drug name: Biphasic insulin lispro

UK brand names: Humulin Mix 30, Humulin Mix 50

Average doses:

- By subcutaneous injection: administer up to 15 minutes before food or shortly after according to requirements

What form does it come in: Suspension for injection including insulin pen refills

Does it interact with other medicines: Yes, the following interactions are known:

- As insulin.

Drug group: Insulins – long acting

Drug name: Insulin degludec (recombinant human insulin analogue – long acting)

UK brand names: Tresiba

Average doses:

- By subcutaneous injection to be given according to requirements

What form does it come in: Solution for injection including insulin pen refills

Does it interact with other medicines: Yes, the following interactions are known:

- As insulin.

Drug name: Insulin degludec with liraglutide

UK brand names: Xultophy

Average doses:

- By subcutaneous injection: when added in addition to oral antidiabetics in type 2 diabetes, initially 10 dose steps daily up to 50 dose steps daily maximum. When transferring from basal insulin in addition to oral antidiabetics in type 2 diabetes, initially 16 dose steps daily

What form does it come in: Solution for injection

Does it interact with other medicines: Yes, the following interactions are known:

- As insulin.
- Some orally administered drugs such as antibiotics and gastro-resistant drugs should be administered 1 hour before or 4 hours after injection.

Drug name: Insulin glarcine (recombinant human insulin analogue – long acting)

UK brand names: Abasaglar, Lantus, Semglee, Toujeo

Average doses:

- By subcutaneous injection according to requirements

(Continued)

What form does it come in: Solution for injection including insulin pen refills

Does it interact with other medicines: Yes, the following interactions are known:

- As insulin.

Drug name: Insulin glarcine with liraglutide

UK brand names: Suliqua

Average doses:

- Depending on previous treatment initially 10 to 30 dose steps up to 60 dose steps (to be administered with metformin)

What form does it come in: Solution for injection (2 different dose strengths)

Does it interact with other medicines: Yes, the following interactions are known:

- As insulin.
- Some orally administered drugs such as antibiotics and gastro-resistant drugs should be administered 1 hour before or 4 hours after injection.

DRUG GROUPS/CONCEPT: BLOOD GLUCOSE LOWERING DRUGS

Blood glucose-lowering drugs are generally used in type 2 diabetes as many require insulin to be produced by the pancreas which does not occur in type 1 diabetes.

Biguanides reduce the production of glucose by the liver, increase the uptake and utilisation of glucose in skeletal muscle. They also reduce the absorption of carbohydrates from the intestines, increase fatty acid oxidation and reduce blood levels of very low-density and low-density cholesterol (Ritter et al., 2020). Alpha glucosidase inhibitors act to delay the digestion of carbohydrates thus reducing blood glucose levels after a meal.

Sulphonylureas act by stimulating the beta cells of the pancreas to produce insulin regardless of glucose levels.

Glucagon-like peptide-1 (GLP1) receptor agonists mimic the action of GLP1 which acts to increase the first phase of insulin release after food, increase the feeling of satiety, reduce gastric emptying and suppress glucagon release (Ashelford et al., 2019). Diabetic Ketoacidosis has been reported with GLP1 receptor antagonists with insulin in type 2 diabetic patients, especially if the insulin is withdrawn (Joint Formulary Committee, 2024).

Dipetidylpeptidase-4 inhibitors (gliptins) also act on the pancreas to increase insulin release by inhibiting the breakdown of GLP1 but as this is glucose-dependent it reduces the risk of hypoglycaemia compared to sulphonylureas (Ritter et al., 2020).

Meglitinides (repaglinide) act in a similar way to the sulphonylureas although they have a more rapid and shorter action and again are less likely to cause hypoglycaemia (Ritter et al., 2020).

Thiazolidinediones (glitazones) reduce blood glucose by increasing the sensitivity of fat and muscle cells to insulin, increasing the uptake of glucose (Willihnganz et al., 2020). However, in recent years there has been concern that these drugs can have serious adverse effects such as heart failure, oedema, weight gain and bone fractures (Ritter et al., 2020).

Selective glucose co-transporter 2 inhibitors promote the excretion of glucose in the urine resulting in glucosuria and increased water and salt loss. This can also have the benefit of reducing blood pressure (Ritter et al., 2020). However several serious complications have been associated with these drugs, including diabetic ketoacidosis in patients with only moderately elevated blood glucose and increased risk of lower limb amputation and Fornier's gangrene (Joint Formulary Committee, 2024).

Drug group: Alpha glucosidase inhibitors

Drug name: Acarbose

UK brand names: None

Average doses:

- Initially 50 mg per day increasing to a maximum of 200 mg three times a day

What form does it come in: Tablet

Does it interact with other medicines: Yes, the following interactions are known:

- Other antidiabetic drugs increase risk of hypoglycaemia.
- Acarbose increases the concentration of digoxin
- Pancreatin decreases the effects of acarbose

Drug group: Biguanides

Drug name: Metformin hydrochloride

UK brand names: Diagemet XL, Glucient SR, Glucophage, Glucophage SR, Meijumet, Metabet SR, Metuxtan SR, Sukkarto, SR, Yaltormin SR

Average doses:

- Initially 500 mg daily increasing up to maximum of 2 grams per day

(Continued)

What form does it come in: Modified release tablet, tablet

Does it interact with other medicines: Yes, the following interactions are known:

- Other antidiabetic drugs increase risk of hypoglycaemia.
- Alcohol (heavy consumption) increases the risk of lactic acidosis.
- The following drugs increase exposure to / concentration or effect of metformin: bictegravir, dolutegravir, fenfluramine, guanfacine, cimetidine, mexiletine, pilostat, ribociclib, risdiplam vantetanib.

Drug group: Dipetidylpeptidase-4 inhibitors (gliptins)

Drug name: Aloglyptin

UK brand names: Vipidia

Average doses:

- 25 mg per day

What form does it come in: Tablet

Does it interact with other medicines: Yes, the following interactions are known:

- Other antidiabetic drugs increase risk of hypoglycaemia.

Drug name: Aloglyptin with metformin

UK brand names: Vipdomet

Average doses:

- 1 tablet twice a day

What form does it come in: Tablet

Does it interact with other medicines: Yes, the following interactions are known:

- As metformin.

Drug name: Linagliptin

UK brand names: Trajenta

Average doses:

- 5 mg per day

What form does it come in: Tablet

Does it interact with other medicines: Yes, the following interactions are known:

- Other antidiabetic drugs increase risk of hypoglycaemia.
- The following drugs decrease exposure to linagliptin: antiandrogens, antiepileptics, mitotane, rifamycins.
- Linagliptin increases exposure to lomitapide.

Drug name: Linaglyptin with metformin

UK brand names: Jentadueto

Average doses:

- 1 tablet twice daily

What form does it come in: Tablet

Does it interact with other medicines: Yes, the following interactions are known:

- As metformin.
- As linaglyptin.

Drug name: Saxaglyptin

UK brand names: Onglyza

Average doses:

- 5 mg per day

What form does it come in: Tablet

(Continued)

Does it interact with other medicines: Yes, the following interactions are known:

- Other antidiabetic drugs increase risk of hypoglycaemia.
- The following drugs increase exposure to saxaglyptin by reducing metabolism: antifungals (azoles), dronedarone, calcium channel blockers (diltiazem, verapamil), cobicistat, crizotinib, grapefruit juice, HIV-protease inhibitors, idealisib, imatinib, levermovir, lomitapide, macrolides, neurokinin-1 receptor antagonists (aprepitant, netupitant).
- The following drugs decrease exposure to saxaglyptin by reducing metabolism: antiandrogens, antiepileptics, mitotane, milotane, rifamycins.

Drug name: Saxaglyptin with metformin

UK brand names: Komboglyze

Average doses:

- 1 tablet twice daily

What form does it come in: Tablet

Does it interact with other medicines: Yes, the following interactions are known:

- As saxaglyptin.
- As metformin.

Drug name: Sitaglyptin

UK brand names: Januvia

Average doses:

- 100 mg per day

What form does it come in: Tablet

Does it interact with other medicines: Yes, the following interactions are known:

- Other antidiabetic drugs increase risk of hypoglycaemia.

Drug name: Sitaglyptin with metformin

UK brand names: Janumet

Average doses:

- 1 tablet twice daily

What form does it come in: Tablet

Does it interact with other medicines: Yes, the following interactions are known:

- As metformin.

Drug name: Vildaglyptin

UK brand names: Galvus

Average doses:

- 50-100 mg per day

What form does it come in: Tablet

Does it interact with other medicines: Yes, the following interactions are known:

- Other antidiabetic drugs increase risk of hypoglycaemia.

Drug name: Vildaglyptin with metformin

UK brand names: Eucreas

Average doses:

- 1 tablet twice a day

What form does it come in: Tablet

Does it interact with other medicines: Yes, the following interactions are known:

- As metformin.

Drug group: Glucagon-like peptide-1 receptor agonists

Drug name: Dulaglutide

UK brand names: Trulicity

Average doses:

- 0.75-1.5 mg weekly by subcutaneous injection up to 4.5 mg maximum per week

What form does it come in: Solution for injection

Does it interact with other medicines: Yes, the following interactions are known:

- Other antidiabetic drugs increase risk of hypoglycaemia.

Drug name: Exenatide

UK brand names: Byetta, Bydureon

Average doses:

- Immediate release subcutaneous injection: 5-10 mg twice a day within 1 hour of main meal. Modified release by subcutaneous injection 2 mg weekly

What form does it come in: Solution for injection, powder and solvent for prolonged release suspension for injection

Does it interact with other medicines: Yes, the following interactions are known:

- Other antidiabetic drugs increase risk of hypoglycaemia.
- Some orally administered drugs such as antibiotics and gastro-resistant drugs should be administered 1 hour before or 4 hours after injection.

Drug name: Liraglutide

UK brand names: Saxenda, Victoza

Average doses:

- 0.6-1.8 mg daily by subcutaneous injection (maximum dose of Saxenda 3 mg per day)

What form does it come in: Solution for injection

Does it interact with other medicines: Yes, the following interactions are known:

- Other antidiabetic drugs increase risk of hypoglycaemia.

Drug name: Lixisenatide

UK brand names: Lyxumia

Average doses:

- 10-20 micrograms per day by subcutaneous injection

What form does it come in: Solution for injection

Does it interact with other medicines: Yes, the following interactions are known:

- As exenatide.

Drug name: Semaglutide

UK brand names: Rybelsus, Wegovy, Ozempic

Average doses:

- 0.25-1 mg weekly by subcutaneous injection. Orally 3-14 mg daily

What form does it come in: Solution for injection, tablet

Does it interact with other medicines: Yes, the following interactions are known:

- Other antidiabetic drugs increase risk of hypoglycaemia.

Drug group: Meglitinides

Drug name: Repaglinide

UK brand names: Enyglid, Prandin

Average doses:

- 500 micrograms to 4 mg before main meals, adjusted to response. Maximum 16 mg per day

(Continued)

What form does it come in: Tablet

Does it interact with other medicines: Yes, the following interactions are known:

- Other antidiabetic drugs increase risk of hypoglycaemia.
- The following drugs increase exposure to repaglinide by reducing metabolism: antifungals (azoles), ciclosporin, clopidogrel, cobicistat, fibrates, filgotinib, HIV-protease inhibitors, idealisib, iron chelators, leflunomide, levermovir, macrolides, opicapone, teriflunomide, trimethoprim.
- The following drugs decrease exposure to repaglinide by reducing metabolism: antiandrogens, antiepileptics, mitotane, pitolisant, rifamycins.

Drug group: Selective glucose co-transporter 2 inhibitors

Drug name: Canagliflozin

UK brand names: Invokana

Average doses:

- 100–300 mg per day

What form does it come in: Tablet

Does it interact with other medicines: Yes, the following interactions are known:

- Other antidiabetic drugs increase risk of hypoglycaemia.
- Rifamycins reduce the effect of canagliflozin

Drug name: Canagliflozin with metformin

UK brand names: Vokanamet

Average doses:

- 1 tablet twice daily

What form does it come in: Tablet

Does it interact with other medicines: Yes, the following interactions are known:

- As canagliflozin.
- As metformin.

Drug name: Dapagliflozin

UK brand names: Forxiga

Average doses:

- 5-10 mg per day

What form does it come in: Tablet

Does it interact with other medicines: Yes, the following interactions are known:

- Other antidiabetic drugs increase risk of hypoglycaemia.

Drug name: Dapagliflozin with metformin

UK brand names: Xigduo

Average doses:

- 1 tablet twice a day

What form does it come in: Tablet

Does it interact with other medicines: Yes, the following interactions are known:

- As metformin.

Drug name: Empagliflozin

UK brand names: Jardiance

Average doses:

- 10-25 mg per day

(Continued)

What form does it come in: Tablet

Does it interact with other medicines: Yes, the following interactions are known:

- Other antidiabetic drugs increase risk of hypoglycaemia.

Drug name: Empagliflozin with linagliptin

UK brand names: Glyxambi

Average doses:

- 10/5-25/5 mg per day (10mg of Empagliflozin with 5mg linagliptin to 25 mg Empagliflozin with 5mg of linagliptin)

What form does it come in: Tablet

Does it interact with other medicines: Yes, the following interactions are known:

- As linaglyptin.

Drug name: Empagliflozin with metformin

UK brand names: Synjardy

Average doses:

- 5/850-12.5/1000 mg twice a day (5mg of Empagliflozin with 850 mg metformin to 12.5 mg Empagliflozin with 1000mg of metformin)

What form does it come in: Tablet

Does it interact with other medicines: Yes, the following interactions are known:

- As metformin.

Drug name: Ertugliflozin

UK brand names: Steglaro

Average doses:

- 5-15 mg per day

What form does it come in: Tablet

Does it interact with other medicines: Yes, the following interactions are known:

- Other antidiabetic drugs increase risk of hypoglycaemia.

Drug group: Sulphonylureas

Drug name: Gliclazide

UK brand names: None

Average doses:

- 40-320 mg per day

What form does it come in: Modified release tablet, tablet

Does it interact with other medicines: Yes, the following interactions are known:

- Other antidiabetic drugs and fibrates increase risk of hypoglycaemia.
- The following drugs increase the concentration or actions of gliclazide: amiodarone, antifungals (azoles),chloramphenicol, clarythromycin, sulfonamides
- The following drugs decrease the concentration or actions of gliclazide: rifamycins

Drug name: Glimepiride

UK brand names: None

Average doses:

- 1-4 mg per day, maximum dose 6 mg per day

What form does it come in: Tablet

Does it interact with other medicines: Yes, the following interactions are known:

- As gliclazide.

The following drug increase the concentration or action of glimepiride: nitisinone

(Continued)

Drug name: Glipizide

UK brand names: None

Average doses:

- 2.5-15 mg per day, maximum dose 20 mg per day

What form does it come in: Tablet

Does it interact with other medicines: Yes, the following interactions are known:

- As gliclazide.

Drug name: Tolbutamide

UK brand names: None

Average doses:

- 0.5-2 grams per day

What form does it come in: Tablet

Does it interact with other medicines: Yes, the following interactions are known:

- As glimepiride.

Drug group: Thiazolidinediones (glitazones)

Drug name: Pioglitazone

UK brand names: Actos, Glidipion

Average doses:

- 15-45 mg per day

What form does it come in: Tablet

Does it interact with other medicines: Yes, the following interactions are known:

- Other antidiabetic drugs increase risk of hypoglycaemia.
- The following drugs increase exposure to pioglitazone by reducing metabolism: antifungals (azoles), clopidogrel, fibrates, iron chelators, leflunomide, opicapone, teriflunomide, trimethoprim.
- The following drugs decrease exposure to pioglitazone by reducing metabolism: rifamycins.

Drug name: Piogliazone with metformin

UK brand names: Competact

Average doses:

- 1 tablet twice a day

What form does it come in: Tablet

Does it interact with other medicines: Yes, the following interactions are known:

- As pioglitazone.
- As metformin.

DRUG GROUPS/CONCEPT: DRUGS TO TREAT THYROID DISORDERS

Drugs within this group aim to either replace missing thyroid hormones or to act to reduce thyroid hormone release or action. Both carbimazole and propylthiouracil act to block the action of the enzyme thyroperoxidase which is involved in the production of thyroid hormones (NICE, 2021). Carbimazole is the first-choice drug as it acts quicker, is cheaper and has fewer side effects, unless pregnancy is considered. In Grave's disease a course of 12–18 months is usually required, however in other conditions anti-thyroid drugs may be considered prior to radioactive iodine or surgery. Lugol's iodine is reserved for short-term use in thyrotoxicosis prior to surgery. It reduces the size and vascularity of the thyroid gland (Ritter et al., 2020) and therefore may reduce surgical complications. Beta blockers are also used in thyrotoxicosis (see Chapter 6).

Levothyroxine and Liothyronine are synthetic versions of thyroxine (T4) and triiodo-thyronine (T3) respectively and therefore replace missing hormones in hypothyroidism, usually for life. Levothyroxine is usually the first line drug of choice with Liothyronine being reserved for emergency use as it has a faster onset and shorter duration of action (Ritter et al., 2020). Treatment of hypothyroidism affects both insulin sensitivity and secretion of insulin from the pancreas and therefore can affect diabetic blood glucose control.

Drug group: Anti-thyroid drugs – sulphur-containing imidazoles

Drug name: Carbimazole

UK brand names: None

Average doses:

- 15–60 mg per day

What form does it come in: Tablet

Does it interact with other medicines: Yes, the following interactions are known:

- Carbimazole increases the concentration or action of the following drugs: digoxinerythromycin, theophylline
- Carbimazole decreases the action or concentration of the following drugs: metyrapone, prednisolone

Drug group: Anti-thyroid drugs – thiouracils

Drug name: Propylthiouracil

UK brand names: None

Average doses:

- 50–400 mg per day

What form does it come in: Tablet

Does it interact with other medicines: Yes, the following interactions are known:

- Metyrapone decreases the effect of propylthiouracil

Drug group: Vitamin and trace elements

Drug name: Iodide with iodine

UK brand names: Lugol's Solution, Aqueous Iodine Oral Solution

Average doses:

- 0.1-0.3 ml, three times per day

What form does it come in: Oral solution

Does it interact with other medicines: No

Drug group: Thyroid hormones

Drug name: Levothyroxine sodium

UK brand names: Eltroxin, Tirosint

Average doses:

- 50-200 micrograms per day

What form does it come in: Tablet

Does it interact with other medicines: Yes, the following interactions are known:

- The following drugs reduce the absorption or effect of levothyroxine: oral antacids, oral calcium salts, proton pump inhibitors oral iron, lanthanum, sucralfate, orlistat.
- The following drugs reduce the effects or concentration of levothyroxine: antiepileptics, ritonavir, amiodarone, sertraline, beta blockers, oestrogens, androgens, corticosteroids, barbiturates.
- Levothyroxine increases the effects of the following drugs: warfarin, digoxin, tricyclic antidepressants.

Drug name: Liothyronine sodium

UK brand names: Cytomel

Average doses:

- 10-60 micrograms per day orally, 5-20 micrograms every 4-12 hours by slow intravenous injection for hypothyroid coma

(Continued)

What form does it come in: Tablet, powder for solution for injection

Does it interact with other medicines: Yes, the following interactions are known:

- The following drugs reduce the absorption of liothyronine: oral antacids, oral iron, lanthanum, sucralfate.
- The following drugs reduce the effects or concentration of liothyronine: antiepileptics, amiodarone, sertraline, beta blockers, oestrogens, androgens, corticosteroids, barbiturates.
- Liothyronine increases the effects of the following drugs: warfarin, digoxin, tricyclic antidepressants (amitriptyline, imipramine).

DRUG GROUPS/CONCEPT: DRUGS FOR CUSHING'S SYNDROME AND DISEASE

Cushing's syndrome can be treated by removing exogenous corticosteroids, surgery, radiotherapy or cortisol-inhibiting drugs, depending on the cause. For the purpose of this book, the medications used will be reviewed.

Ketoconazole inhibits a number of enzymes preventing the production of cortisol as well as inhibiting cholesterol and aldosterone synthesis. It also has an effect on the production of androgens which can be useful in females with hirsutism, but reduces libido and can cause gynaecomastia in men. Ketoconazole may also have a direct effect on corticotropic tumour cells in patients with Cushing's disease (Datapharm, 2023). Ketoconazole is also an antifungal drug as discussed in Chapter 2, along with the numerous drug interactions that occur.

Metyrapone specifically inhibits 11β hydroxylase enzyme in the adrenal cortex reducing the production of cortisol. This leads to an increase in the production of adrenocorticotrophic hormone which means that metyrapone can also be used to test the function of the anterior pituitary gland (Joint Formulary Committee, 2024).

Drug group: Enzyme inhibitors

Drug name: Ketoconazole

UK brand names: None

Average doses:

- 400–800 mg per day

What form does it come in: Tablet

Does it interact with other medicines: Yes, the following interactions are known:

- See ketoconazole in Chapter 2.

Drug name: Metyrapone

UK brand names: Metopirone

Average doses:

- 0.25–6 grams per day

What form does it come in: Capsule

Does it interact with other medicines: Yes, the following interactions are known:

- The following drugs reduce the effect of metyrapone: antiepileptics, cyproheptadine, carbimazole, combined oral contraceptives, chlorpromazine, propylthiouracil, amitriptyline.

DRUG GROUPS/CONCEPT: DRUGS TO TREAT ADDISON'S DISEASE

In Addison's disease, there is a lack of production of hormones from the adrenal cortex. Treatment is therefore hormone replacement. Mineralocorticoid replacement is with fludrocortisone, whereas glucocorticoid replacement is with hydrocortisone. Androgens may need to be replaced in women but this is not discussed in this book.

Drug group: Adrenal corticosteroids

Drug name: Fludrocortisone acetate

UK brand names: None

Average doses:

- 50–300 micrograms per day

(Continued)

What form does it come in: Tablet

Does it interact with other medicines: Yes, the following interactions are known:

- The following drugs increase the effects of fludrocortisone acetate: antifungals, cobicistat, macrolides, HIV protease inhibitors, idelalisib, neurokinin 1 receptor antagonists.
- The following drugs reduce the effect or concentration of fludrocortisone acetate; antiepileptics, mifepristone, mitotane, rifamycins.
- Fludrocortisone acetate reduces the effects of the following drugs: aspirin, mifamurtide, neuromuscular blocking drugs, sodium phenylbutyrate, somatropin, suxamethonium.
- Fludrocortisone acetate increases the risk of gastrointestinal bleeding when given with the following: aspirin, deferasirox, NSAIDs.
- Fludrocortisone acetate increases the risk of immunosuppression when given with monoclonal antibodies and can cause an increased risk of infection with live vaccines.
- Fludrocortisone acetate increases the risk of gastrointestinal perforation when given with nicorandil.

Drug name: Hydrocortisone – see Chapter 2.

DRUGS FOR METABOLIC DISORDERS IN PREGNANCY AND BREASTFEEDING

Good control of metabolism is especially important in pregnancy and during breastfeeding, in particular when it comes to blood glucose. Gestational diabetes can cause serious complications for both the pregnant person and baby, with larger than normal babies, increase risk of stillbirth, premature labour and increased likelihood of the child developing obesity and type 2 diabetes in later life. Increased blood glucose testing is required during pregnancy with an aim to maintain blood glucose control with either oral therapy or insulin without causing hypoglycaemia (NICE, 2020). Insulin does not cross the placenta and therefore it is safe during pregnancy. Metformin is also considered safe in pregnancy and breastfeeding, whereas other oral antidiabetic drugs are to be avoided due to neonatal hypoglycaemia (sulphonylureas) or potential foetal toxicity (Joint Formulary Committee, 2024).

Good thyroid control is also important in pregnancy due to increased risk both to the pregnant person and the foetus, including preeclampsia, pre-term delivery, low birth weight, miscarriage and stillbirth. Levothyroxine dosage requirements will increase in pregnancy as the foetus is reliant on maternal thyroid hormones in the first trimester. Propylthiouracil is preferred in the first trimester with carbimazole in the second and third trimesters due to the relative risks and severity of foetal abnormalities and liver dysfunction. Breastfeeding is considered safe whilst taking anti-thyroid drugs but the dose should be kept to a minimum (Hyer, 2018).

Pregnancy is rare in patients with Cushing's disease as it impairs fertility and increases the likelihood of miscarriage. If medical treatment is required, metyrapone has been most commonly used, although there is a risk of foetal adrenal insufficiency. Ketoconazole has the potential to cause feminisation in male foetuses and should be avoided in the first trimester. It has also been found to be teratogenic and abortogenic in animal studies, although this has not been seen in the small number of women who have taken it in pregnancy (Hamblin et al., 2022). The manufacturers advise avoiding taking either drug whilst breastfeeding (Joint Formulary Committee, 2024).

Glucocorticoid and mineralocorticoid replacement for Addison's disease is safe and essential during pregnancy when increase dosages may be required (Oliveira et al., 2018).

LEARNING FROM A CASE STUDY: TEST YOUR KNOWLEDGE

Meera is a 61-year-old who works part-time as a school cook. She has type 2 diabetes and hypothyroidism and attended her GP for a review. Previously her diabetes had been managed with diet alone but on last review metformin was introduced as her HbA1c was 77mmol/mol. Her BMI is 33 and this has increased in the last year, and she is finding that she is exercising less and less and is feeling very tired. Her QRISK2 is 25%. Her current drug regimen is metformin 1 g twice a day, levothyroxine 50 micrograms daily, atorvastatin 20 mg daily. Her HbA1c is currently 65mmol/mol.

1   What non-pharmaceutical advice would you give to Meera to help with her type 2 diabetes?
2   What do the NICE guidelines suggest would be the next step in Meera's treatment for type 2 diabetes?
3   Are there any drugs that Meera is taking that might affect her blood glucose levels?
4   Looking at Meera's medical history and drug regimen what else might need to be reviewed?

IF I REMEMBER 5 THINGS FROM THIS CHAPTER:

1   Metabolic disorders have an affect across the body.
2   Metabolic disorders affect large numbers of the population and therefore drugs in this chapter will be commonly prescribed.
3   Metabolic disorders require holistic treatment with medication used alongside lifestyle factors.
4   Good control of metabolic conditions is essential in pregnancy.
5   Metabolic conditions can cause medical emergencies and both patients and healthcare professionals need to have education to recognise signs, symptoms and treatments.

ANSWERS TO CASE STUDY QUESTIONS

1   Meera is overweight and reducing her weight might help reduce her blood glucose levels. She may benefit from advice on diet and exercise.
2   Meera's HbA1c is still too high. She is also on a statin which suggests that she has raised blood cholesterol and may be at higher risk of adverse cardiovascular events (QRISK2 is greater than 10%). The NICE guidelines suggest introducing a selective glucose co-transporter 2 inhibitor.
3   Statins can also raise blood glucose levels due to decreased insulin sensitivity, but current guidance suggests that the benefits of reducing cholesterol outweigh the risks. Levothyroxine can also affect blood glucose control and increase the requirements of antidiabetic medication.
4   Given some of Meera's symptoms and her history of hypothyroidism it would be beneficial to check her thyroid function as she may need an increase in levothyroxine. She may also need her blood cholesterol levels checked.

REFERENCES AND RECOMMENDED READING

Ashelford, S., Raynsford, J. and Taylor, V. (2019) *Pathophysiology and Pharmacology in Nursing* (2nd edn). London: Sage Publishing.

Cappola, A.R., Desai, A.S., Medici, M. et al. (2019) Thyroid and cardiovascular disease research agenda for enhancing knowledge, prevention, and treatment. *Circulation*, *139*(25): 2892–2909. www.ahajournals.org/doi/epub/10.1161/CIRCULATIONAHA. 118.036859

Datapharm (2023) Electronic medicines compendium. Available at: www.medicines. org.uk/emc

Diabetes UK (2020) Diabetes prevalence 2019. Available at: www.diabetes.org.uk/ professionals/position-statements-reports/statistics/diabetes-prevalence-2019

Hamblin, R., Coulden, A., Fountas, A. and Karavitaki, N. (2022) The diagnosis and management of Cushing's syndrome in pregnancy. *Journal of Neuroendocrinology*, *34*(8): e13118. doi:10.1111/jne.13118.

Handisurya et al. (2008) Hypothyroidism: Glucose metabolism improves with endocrine therapy. *Nature Clinical Practice Endocrinology & Metabolism*, *4*: 474. https://doi.org/ 10.1038/ncpendmet0904

Hyer, S. (2018) Caring for women with thyroid disorders in pregnancy. *British Journal of Midwifery*, *18*(7): 434–439.

Joint Formulary Committee (2024) British National Formulary. Available at: https://bnf. nice.org.uk/

National Institute for Health and Care Excellence (NICE) (2022a) Type 1 diabetes in adults: Diagnosis and management. Nice guideline [NG17]. Available at: www.nice.org.uk/ guidance/ng17

National Institute for Health and Care Excellence (NICE) (2022b) Type 2 diabetes in adults: Management. Available at: www.nice.org.uk/guidance/ng28/chapter/ Recommendations#hba1c-measurement-and-targets

National Institute for Health and Care Excellence (NICE) (2021) Hyperthyroidism. Available at: https://cks.nice.org.uk/topics/hyperthyroidism/

National Institute for Health and Care Excellence (NICE) (2020) Diabetes in pregnancy: Management from preconception to the postnatal period. Available at: www.nice.org.uk/guidance/ng3/chapter/Recommendations#antenatal-care-for-women-with-diabetes

Oliveira, D., Lages, A., Paiva, S. and Carrilho, F. (2018) Treatment of Addison's disease during pregnancy. *Endocrinology, Diabetes & Metabolism Case Reports*, *17*: 179. https://doi.org/10.1530/EDM-17-0179

Ritter, J.M., Flower, R., Henderson, H., Kong Loke, Y., MacEwan, D. and Rang, H.P. (2020) *Rang and Dale's Pharmacology* (9th edn). Edinburgh: Elsevier.

Seifter, J.L., Walsh, E.C. and Sloane, D.E. (2022) *Integrated Physiology and Pathophysiology*. Philadelphia, PA: Elsevier.

Willihnganz, M.J., Gurevitz, S.L. and Clayton, B.D. (2020) *Clayton's Basic Pharmacology for Nurses*. St Louis: Elsevier.

5 MEDICINES FOR DEGENERATIVE CONDITIONS

RACHAEL MAJOR

AFTER READING THIS CHAPTER YOU WILL BE ABLE TO:

- Discuss the aetiology of degenerative conditions and the implications for treatments.
- Consider the implications of an aging population on degenerative diseases.
- Discuss the pharmaceutical treatment of Parkinson's disease, multiple sclerosis, osteoporosis, macular degeneration and glaucoma.
- Apply knowledge around medicines for degenerative conditions to support clinical decision making.

OVERVIEW

Degenerative diseases are characterised by a progressive loss of function in the body, either an organ, system or more widely. There are many degenerative conditions that occur across the lifespan, with frequency increasing as the population ages. Degenerative diseases can be caused by environmental, lifestyle or genetic factors or a combination, although aging may play a role, along with unknown causes. Whilst this book addresses medicines, for many of the degenerative conditions, changes in lifestyle such as stopping smoking, reducing alcohol consumption, a healthy diet and exercise play an important role in treatment and prevention. Some of the conditions in this category have little effective drug treatment at this point and maintenance of function through physiotherapy and occupational therapy are key as well as psychological, social and financial support.

A number of conditions that are degenerative as also classified in other ways. For example, rheumatoid arthritis is a degenerative disorder caused by an autoimmune condition and drugs treatments for this can be found in Chapter 2. Many cardiovascular conditions may also be classed as degenerative, but their treatment is found in Chapter 6 and metabolic conditions in Chapter 4. Pain is also an important consideration in many of the degenerative conditions and this is addressed in Chapter 7. The most common neurodegenerative condition in the UK is Alzheimer's disease, but this is not within the scope of this book.

This chapter will address drug treatment of Parkinson's disease, the second most common neurodegenerative disease after Alzheimer's in the UK. Parkinson's disease affects 145,000 people in the UK (Parkinson's UK, 2022) with symptoms of tremor, difficulty initiating voluntary movement, muscle rigidity, depression and in some cases dementia.

In the UK, 105,800 people are living with multiple sclerosis (Public Health England 2020), an autoimmune disease that causes progressive loss of myelin and nerve damage in the central nervous system (CNS). For many this is seen over many years with a relapsing remitting pattern of disease initially until moving into a secondary progressive phase, although for some, primary progression occurs with no remission. This chapter will address the drug treatments primarily to suppress or modulate the immune response causing this condition, although drugs for muscle spasm both in multiple sclerosis and motor neuron disease are also included.

Osteoporosis is characterised by low bone density and fragility, increasing the risk of fractures. In 2019 there were 3,775,000 individuals living with osteoporosis in the UK, 78.3% of them women, with osteoporotic fractures costing approximately 2.4% of the UK healthcare spending (International Osteoporosis Foundation and Scope 21, 2021).

Degenerative eye conditions such as age-related macular degeneration and glaucoma also impact on the lives of the population, potentially leading to sight loss. Glaucoma is a group of eye diseases where, in most cases, increased intraocular pressure can lead to damage of the optic nerve. Primary open angle glaucoma becomes more common with age, with about 8% of the population affected at 80 years of age (NICE, 2022a).

Degenerative conditions are not confined to the older population, with genetic factors accounting for most childhood degenerative conditions, such as Duchenne muscular dystrophy. Drugs for childhood disorders are not addressed in this book. Cancers are also a form of degenerative conditions; however, this is a very specialist and ever-changing area and will not be addressed in this book.

GO FURTHER

For cancer drugs Cancer Research UK has an excellent website which can be found here: www.cancerresearchuk.org/about-cancer/treatment/drugs

For dementia drug treatments please see Holland, E. (2022) *The Nurse's Guide to Mental Health Medicines* (2nd edn). London: Sage Publications.

The medicines list

- Drugs for Parkinson's disease
  - Antimuscarinics
  - Catechol-O-methyltransferase (COMT) inhibitors
  - Dopamine precursors
  - Dopaminergic drugs
  - Monoamine oxidase-B inhibitors

- Drugs to treat multiple sclerosis
  - Immunosuppressants
  - Immunostimulants
  - Potassium channel blocker
- Drugs to treat motor neurone disease and symptoms
  - Neuroprotective drugs
  - Anti-malarial
  - Muscle relaxants
- Drugs to treat osteoporosis
  - Bisphosphonates
  - Bone reabsorption inhibitors
  - Parathyroid hormone and analogues
  - Monoclonal antibodies
- Drugs to treat macular degeneration
  - Vascular endothelial growth factor
  - Photosensitisers
- Drugs to treat glaucoma
  - Beta receptor antagonists
  - Carbonic anhydrase inhibitors
  - Parasympathomimetics
  - Prostaglandins and prostamides
  - Alpha adrenoceptor agonists

This section will address the drug treatment for degenerative conditions, very briefly explaining their actions related to the pathophysiology.

DRUG GROUPS/CONCEPT: DRUGS FOR PARKINSON'S DISEASE

Parkinson's disease is caused by the loss of dopaminergic neurons in the substantial nigra of the basal ganglia, an area of the brain responsible for maintaining posture, muscle tone and initiation of voluntary movement. Normally there is a balance between two neurotransmitters in this area, dopamine (which is inhibitory) and acetylcholine (which is excitatory). With the depletion of approximately 80% of dopamine, symptoms of Parkinson's disease occur. Drugs to treat Parkinson's disease try to redress the balance by either reducing acetylcholine or increasing the effect of dopamine. Dopamine cannot cross the blood brain barrier so levodopa is given which can, along with a second drug, either carbidopa or benserazide hydrochloride which are dopa decarboxylase inhibitors. As dopa decarboxylase inhibitors cannot pass through the blood brain barrier, this prevents levodopa being converted into dopamine until it has passed through the blood brain barrier, where it can act on dopamine receptors. Unfortunately, as the disease progresses and more cells are lost, this becomes less effective. Patients report an on/off effect, particularly with levodopa treatment where they have reduced mobility during off periods when the medication has worn off. It is important that patients receive their medication at the prescribed time and that it is not delayed, to help reduce off periods as much as possible. Long-term use of levodopa also causes dyskinesia; rapid, involuntary body movements, which can be particularly difficult for people to manage.

Dopamine receptor agonists also act on the dopamine receptors whilst they are still present in existing cells. Catechol-O-methyltransferase inhibitors (COMT inhibitors) reduce the breakdown of dopamine and therefore more is available to bind to any receptors (Willihnganz et al., 2020). Amantadine has been shown to increase the release of dopamine and reduce dopamine reuptake in cells by inhibiting the effects of the glutamate NMDA receptor (Chang and Ramphul, 2022). Amantadine is also used for fatigue in multiple sclerosis. Parkinson's drugs that increase dopamine (especially dopamine receptor agonists) have also been found to increase the risk of impulse control disorders such as gambling, binge eating, obsessive shopping and hypersexuality, especially in those who have a previous history of similar conduct. These drugs can also cause excessive sleepiness, hallucinations, depression, postural hypotension and dizziness.

Antimuscarinic drugs reduce the effects of acetylcholine and therefore help to reduce tremor. Antimuscarinic drugs cause side effects such as dry mouth, nausea, blurred vision and urinary retention.

Mono-amine oxidase B inhibitors have been found to have two effects. Firstly, they inhibit another enzyme that breaks down dopamine, monoamine oxidase, and therefore increase the amount of dopamine available. There is also some evidence that some MAO-B inhibitors may be neuroprotective and therefore reduce the loss of dopaminergic cells and slow the progression of Parkinson's (Ritter et al., 2020).

Drug group: Antimuscarinics (anticholinergics)

Drug name: Orphenadrine hydrochloride

UK brand names: None

Average doses:

- 150–300 mg per day

What form does it come in: Oral solution

Does it interact with other medicines: Yes, the following interactions are known:

- May enhance the effects of other anti-muscarinic drugs.
- May reduce gastric motility which may reduce absorption of other orally administered drugs.

(Continued)

Drug name: Procyclidine hydrochloride

UK brand names: Kemadrin

Average doses:

- 2.5–30 mg per day

What form does it come in: Solution for injection, oral solution, tablet

Does it interact with other medicines: Yes, the following interactions are known:

- As orphenadrine.
- Paroxetine significantly increases plasma levels of procyclidine.

Drug name: Trihexyphenidyl hydrochloride (benhexol hydrochloride)

UK brand names: None

Average doses:

- 2–15 mg per day

What form does it come in: Oral solution, tablet

Does it interact with other medicines: Yes, the following interactions are known:

- As orphenadrine.

Drug group: Catechol-O-methyltransferase (COMT) inhibitors

Drug name: Entacapone

UK brand names: Comtess

Average doses:

- 200 mg with every dose of levodopa with dopa-decarboxylase inhibitor

What form does it come in: Tablet

Does it interact with other medicines: Yes, the following interactions are known:

- Increases exposure to levodopa and methyldopa.
- Increases cardiovascular risks when given with sympathomimetics (adrenaline, epinephrine, inotropes).
- Increases blood pressure when given with irreversible monoamine oxidase inhibitors.

Drug name: Opicapone

UK brand names: Ongentys

Average doses:

- 50 mg per day

What form does it come in: Tablet

Does it interact with other medicines: Yes, the following interactions are known:

- As entacapone.
- Increases exposure to loperamide, moclobemide and montelukast.

Drug name: Tolcapone

UK brand names: Tasmar

Average doses:

- 100-200 mg, three times per day

What form does it come in: Tablet

Does it interact with other medicines: Yes, the following interactions are known:

- As entacapone.

Drug group: Dopamine precursors

Drug name: Co-beneldopa

UK brand names: Madopar

Average doses:

- Immediate release: 50-200 mg, 3-4 times per day; modified release: 1-2 capsules, three times a day

What form does it come in: Dispersible tablet, modified release capsule, capsule

Does it interact with other medicines: Yes, the following interactions are known:

- The following drugs reduce the effects of co-beneldopa: antiepileptics, antipsychotics (2nd generation), benperidol, droperidol, antimuscarinics, flupentixol, haloperidol, iron, isoniazid, metoclopramide, phenothiazines, pimozide, vulpicide, tolcapone, tryptophan, zuclopenthixol.
- The following drugs increase the effect of co-beneldopa: entacapone, monoamine oxidase inhibitors-B, memantine, opicapone, tolcapone.
- The following drugs increase risks of unwanted side effects (some serious) with co-beneldopa: baclofen, linezolid, irreversible monoamine oxidase inhibitors, moclobemide.

Drug name: Co-careldopa

UK brand names: Caremet, Duodopa, Sinemet

Average doses:

- Immediate release: 200/2000 mg per day. Modified release: Caremet 100-200 mg twice daily; Sinemet CR initially 1 tablet twice daily, dose adjusted to response; gel: for specialist use

What form does it come in: Modified release tablet, tablet, gel

Does it interact with other medicines: Yes, the following interactions are known:

- As co-beneldopa.

Drug name: Levodopa with carbidopa and entacapone

UK brand names: Stalevo

Average doses:

* 1 tablet for each dose, 7-10 tablets per day (note many dose variations)

What form does it come in: Tablet

Does it interact with other medicines: Yes, the following interactions are known:

* As co-beneldopa.
* As entacapone.

Drug group: Dopaminergic drugs

Drug name: Amantadine hydrochloride

UK brand names: None

Average doses:

* 100-200 mg twice daily

What form does it come in: Oral solution, capsule

Does it interact with other medicines: Yes, the following interactions are known:

* The following drugs increase exposure to amantadine: memantine.
* The following drugs decrease exposure to amantadine: antipsychotics (2nd generation), benperidol, droperidol, flupentixol, haloperidol, metoclopramide, phenothiazines, pimozide, sulpiride, zuclopenthixol.
* The following drugs increase risks of unwanted side effects (some serious) with amantadine: bupropion, memantine, antimuscarinics.

(Continued)

Drug name: Apomorphine hydrochloride

UK brand names: Apo-go, Dacepton

Average doses:

- By subcutaneous injection: 3–30 mg in divided doses; by subcutaneous infusion: 15–60 micrograms/kg/hour during waking hours

What form does it come in: Solution for injection, solution for infusion

Does it interact with other medicines: Yes, the following interactions are known:

- The following drugs increase exposure to apomorphine: memantine.
- The following drugs decrease exposure to apomorphine: antipsychotics (2nd generation), benperidol, droperidol, flupentixol, haloperidol, metoclopramide, phenothiazines, pimozide, sulpiride, zuclopenthixol.
- The following drugs increase risks of unwanted side effects (some serious) with apomorphine: 5HT3 receptor antagonists (granisetron, palonosetron, ondansetron), bupropion, antimuscarinics, drugs causing hypotension, drugs that prolong the QT interval.

Drug name: Pramipexole

UK brand names: Mirapexin, Oprymea, Pipexus

Average doses:

- Immediate release: maximum 3.3 mg per day in 3 divided doses; modified release: maximum 3.15 mg per day, titrate to response

What form does it come in: Modified release tablet, tablet

Does it interact with other medicines: Yes, the following interactions are known:

- The following drugs increase exposure to pramipexole: memantine, isavuconazole, dolutegravir, amantadine, cimetidine, ranolazine, trimethoprim, vandetanib.
- The following drugs decrease exposure to pramipexole: antipsychotics (2nd generation), benperidol, droperidol, flupentixol, haloperidol, metoclopramide, phenothiazines, pimozide, sulpiride, zuclopenthixol.
- The following drugs increase risks of unwanted side effects (some serious) with pramipexole: bupropion, drugs causing hypotension.

Drug name: Ropinirole

UK brand names: Adartrel, Eppinex, Raponer, Ralnea, ReQuip, Repinex, Ropiqual, Spiroco

Average doses:

- Immediate release: 3-4 mg, three times per day; modified release: 8 mg once per day, maximum 24 mg per day

What form does it come in: Modified release tablet, tablet

Does it interact with other medicines: Yes, the following interactions are known:

- The following drugs increase exposure to ropinirole: memantine, mexiletine, fluvoxamine.
- The following drugs decrease exposure to ropinirole: antipsychotics (2nd generation), benperidol, droperidol, flupentixol, haloperidol, metoclopramide, phenothiazines, pimozide, sulpiride, zuclopenthixol, hormone replacement therapy.
- The following drugs increase risks of unwanted side effects (some serious) with ropinirole: drugs causing hypotension.

Drug name: Rotigotine

UK brand names: Neupro

Average doses:

- 2-16 mg per day

What form does it come in: Transdermal patch

Does it interact with other medicines: Yes, the following interactions are known:

- The following drugs increase exposure to rotigotine: memantine.
- The following drugs decrease exposure to rotigotine: antipsychotics (2nd generation), benperidol, droperidol, flupentixol, haloperidol, metoclopramide, phenothiazines, pimozide, sulpiride, zuclopenthixol.
- The following drugs increase risks of unwanted side effects (some serious) with rotigotine: drugs causing hypotension.

Drug group: Monoamine oxidase-B inhibitors

Drug name: Rasagline

UK brand names: Azilect

Average doses:

- 1 mg per day

What form does it come in: Tablet

Does it interact with other medicines: Yes, the following interactions are known:

- The following drugs increase exposure to rasagline: combined hormonal contraceptives, mexiletine, moclobemide, ciprofloxacin.
- The following drugs increase risks of unwanted side effects (some serious including hypertensive crisis) with rasagline: amphetamines, beta 2 antagonists, bupropion, linezolid, monoamine oxidase inhibitors (irreversible), methylphenidate, pethidine, ozanimod, reboxetine, soiriamfetol, sympathomimetics (inotropes, vasoconstrictors).
- In combination with drugs that can cause bradycardia, hypotension, serotonin syndrome, these side effects are more likely.

Drug name: Safinamide

UK brand names: Xadago

Average doses:

- 50-100 mg per day

What form does it come in: Tablet

Does it interact with other medicines: Yes, the following interactions are known:

- The following drugs increase risks of unwanted side effects (some serious including hypertensive crisis) with safinamide: amphetamines, beta 2 antagonists, bupropion, linezolid, monoamine oxidase inhibitors (irreversible), methylphenidate, pethidine, ozanimod, reboxetine, soiriamfetol, sympathomimetics (inotropes, vasoconstrictors).
- In combination with drugs that can cause bradycardia, hypotension, serotonin syndrome, these side effects are more likely.

Drug name: Selegiline hydrochloride

UK brand names: Eldepryl

Average doses:

- 5-10 mg per day

What form does it come in: Tablet

Does it interact with other medicines: Yes, the following interactions are known:

- Food high in tyramine such as mature cheese, salami, pickled herring, beef and yeast extracts, fermented soya bean extract, some beers, lagers and wines should be avoided as they can cause hypertension with selegiline.
- The following drugs increase exposure to selegiline: combined hormonal contraceptives, moclobemide, hormone replacement therapy.
- The following drugs increase risks of unwanted side effects (some serious including hypertensive crisis) with selegiline: amphetamines, beta 2 antagonists, bupropion, linezolid, monoamine oxidase inhibitors (irreversible), methylphenidate, pethidine, ozanimod, reboxetine, soiriamfetol, sympathomimetics (inotropes, vasoconstrictors).
- In combination with drugs that can cause bradycardia, hypotension, serotonin syndrome, these side effects are more likely.

DRUG GROUPS/CONCEPT: DRUGS TO TREAT MULTIPLE SCLEROSIS

Multiple sclerosis is an autoimmune disorder causing destruction of the myelin and nerve cells within the CNS. Many of the drugs used in the treatment of multiple sclerosis are designed to modulate the immune response to reduce further damage to nerve cells and are used in relapsing remitting multiple sclerosis. Interferon beta is an anti-inflammatory cytokine or cell messenger which reduces activity of a number of cells within the inflammatory response including lymphocytes, antibodies and T cells. Glatiramer acetate induces the production of Th2 cells which produce anti-inflammatory cytokines (Wei et al., 2021) and the action of dimethyl fumerate is not fully understood.

Monoclonal antibodies have also now been introduced to selectively act against B lymphocytes and/or T lymphocytes, reducing their proliferation, effects and in some cases their ability to get into the CNS. They are also associated with an increased risk of developing other autoimmune disorders, as well an infection. Teriflunomide inhibits the enzyme pyrimidine synthase which reduces the proliferation of B and T lymphocytes (Wei et al., 2021).

Fingolimod, ozanimod and siponimod all act by preventing lymphocytes from leaving the lymph nodes and reducing T cells from entering the CNS (Datapharm 2023). Both ozanimod and siponimod are also thought to promote myelin regeneration (Wei et al., 2021) although they are currently not recommended by NICE (2022b).

Other treatments for multiple sclerosis focus on managing symptoms – for example fampridine, a potassium channel blocker, has been found to improve walking speed; muscle relaxants such as baclofen and cannabinoids are used to reduce spasm; corticosteroids such as methylprednisolone are used during a relapse to reduce inflammation (see Chapter 2); and analgesics for pain (see Chapter 7).

Drug group: Potassium channel blockers

Drug name: Fampridine

UK brand names: Fampyra

Average doses:

- 10 mg every 12 hours

What form does it come in: Modified release capsule

Does it interact with other medicines: Yes, the following interactions are known:

- Cimetidine increases the concentration of fampridine.

Drug group: Immunostimulants – interferons

Drug name: Interferon beta

UK brand names: Avonex, Rebif, Betaferon, Extavia

Average doses:

- Different brands have different dosages; dose give every other day to three times per week

What form does it come in: Solution for injection, powder and solvent for solution for injection

Does it interact with other medicines: Yes, the following interactions are known:

- Increases exposure to aminophylline and theophylline.
- Increases effect of other myelosuppressants.

Drug name: Peginterferon beta-1a

UK brand names: Plegridy

Average doses:

- Tritated up to 125 micrograms every two weeks

What form does it come in: Solution for injection

Does it interact with other medicines: Yes, the following interactions are known:

- As interferon beta.

Drug group: Immunostimulants – other

Drug name: Glatiramer acetate

UK brand names: Brabio, Copaxone

Average doses:

- 20 mg per day or 40 mg three times a week

What form does it come in: Solution for injection

Does it interact with other medicines: No

Drug group: Immunosuppressants – immunomodulating drugs

Drug name: Dimethyl fumerate

UK brand names: Tecfidera, Skilarence (for psoriasis, dose not included here)

Average doses:

- 120–240 mg twice a day

(Continued)

What form does it come in: Gastro-resistant capsule

Does it interact with other medicines: Yes, the following interactions are known:

- Excessive consumption of alcohol increases adverse gastrointestinal effects.
- Avoid live vaccines – increased risk of infection.

Drug name: Fingolimod

UK brand names: Gilenya

Average doses:

- 500 micrograms per day

What form does it come in: Capsule

Does it interact with other medicines: Yes, the following interactions are known:

- The following drugs increase exposure to fingolimod: diltiazem, verapamil.
- The following drugs decrease exposure to fingolimod: antiandrogens, antiepileptics, mitotane, St John's Wort.
- Avoid live vaccines – increased risk of infection.

Drug name: Ozanimod

UK brand names: Zeposia

Average doses:

- 0.92 mg per day (titrated to this dose over two weeks)

What form does it come in: Tablet

Does it interact with other medicines: Yes, the following interactions are known:

- Tyramine rich food increase the risk of hypertensive crisis.
- The following drugs increase exposure to ozanimod: ciclosporin, clopidogrel, eltrombopag, fibrates, leflunomide.
- The following drugs decrease exposure to ozanimod: MAO-B inhibitors, rifamycin.

- The following drugs increase risks of unwanted side effects (some serious including hypertensive crisis) with ozanimod: linezolid, MAO-B inhibitors, MAO inhibitors (irreversible), opioids, moclobemide, SSRIs, sympathomimetics (vasoconstrictors), tricyclic antidepressants.
- Avoid live vaccines – increased risk of infection.
- Increased risk of immunosuppression with alemtuzumab.

Drug name: Ponesimod

UK brand names: Ponvory

Average doses:

- 20 mg per day (titrate to this dose over 2 weeks)

What form does it come in: Capsule

Does it interact with other medicines: Yes, the following interactions are known:

- Increased level of immunosuppression when given with other immunosuppressants.
- May reduce effectiveness of vaccines.
- Avoid live vaccines – increased risk of infection.

Drug name: Siponimod

UK brand names: Mayzent

Average doses:

- 1-2 mg per day

What form does it come in: Tablet

Does it interact with other medicines: Yes, the following interactions are known:

- The following drugs increase exposure to siponimod: amiodarone, antifungals, cobicistat, HIV-protease inhibitors, idelalisib, clarithromycin.
- The following drugs decrease exposure to siponimod: antiandrogens, bosentan, mitotane NNRTIs, rifamycin, St John's Wort.
- Avoid live vaccines – increased risk of infection.
- Increased risk of immunosuppression with alemtuzumab.

Drug group: Immunosuppressants – monoclonal antibodies – anti-lymphocyte

Drug name: Alemtuzumab

UK brand names: Lemtrada

Average doses:

- 12 mg per day for 3-5 days every 12 months

What form does it come in: Solution for infusion

Does it interact with other medicines: Yes, the following interactions are known:

- Ozanimod and Siponimod increase immunosuppression.
- Increased level of immunosuppression when given with other immunosuppressants.
- May reduce effectiveness of vaccines.
- Avoid live vaccines – increased risk of infection.

Drug name: Natalizumab

UK brand names: Tysabri

Average doses:

- 300 mg every four weeks

What form does it come in: Solution for infusion

Does it interact with other medicines: Yes, the following interactions are known:

- Increased level of immunosuppression when given with other immunosuppressants.
- May reduce effectiveness of vaccines.
- Avoid live vaccines – increased risk of infection.

Drug name: Ocrelizumab

UK brand names: Ocrevus

Average doses:

- 600 mg every six months

What form does it come in: Solution for infusion

Does it interact with other medicines: Yes, the following interactions are known:

- As natalizuma.

Drug name: Ofatumumab

UK brand names: Kesimpta

Average doses:

- 20 mg once a month

What form does it come in: Solution for injection (in prefilled pen)

Does it interact with other medicines: Yes, the following interactions are known:

- As natalizumab.

Drug group: Immunosuppressants – pyrimidine synthesis inhibitors

Drug name: Teriflunomide

UK brand names: Aubagio

Average doses:

- 14 mg per day

What form does it come in: Tablet

Does it interact with other medicines: Yes, the following interactions are known:

- Teriflunomide increases exposure to the following drugs: aripiprazole, risperidone, atomoxetine, galantamine, metoprolol, nebivolol, darifenacin, eliglustat, mexiletine, SSRIs, tetrabenazine, tricyclic antidepressants, vortioxetine.
- Teriflunomide decreases the efficacy of the following drugs: codeine, tramadol, tamoxifen.
- The following drugs decrease exposure to teriflunomide: rifamycin.

DRUG GROUPS/CONCEPT: DRUGS TO TREAT MOTOR NEURONE DISEASE

There is very little treatment for motor neurone disease available, with other drugs used for symptom control only. Riluzole is thought to inhibit glutamate-associated cell death in the CNS and it has been found to extend life for a few months in clinical trials (Datapharm, 2023). NICE (2019) recommends quinine as the first level treatment for muscle cramps with baclofen if this is not effective. Tizanidine, dantrolene or gabapentin (see Chapter 7) are alternative options. Quinine is an antimalarial drug but it also reduces excitability in motor nerves, reducing muscle contractions. Baclofen is a selective GABAB receptor agonist which works in the CNS where it inhibits motor neurones and therefore reduces muscle spasms (Ritter et al., 2020). Tizanidine also acts in the CNS, reducing the release of glutamine and aspartate, which again inhibits motor neurone activity. Dantrolene acts on skeletal muscle cells to reduce influx of calcium, again reducing muscle contractions (Joint Formulary Committee, 2024).

Drug group: Neuroprotective drugs

Drug name: Riluzole

UK brand names: Teglutik, Rilutek

Average doses:

- 50 mg twice a day

What form does it come in: Oral suspension, tablet

Does it interact with other medicines: Yes, the following interactions are known:

- Chargrilled food decreases exposure to riluzole.
- The following drugs increase exposure to riluzole: ciprofloxacin, fluvoxamine.

Drug group: Anti-malarial

Drug name: Quinine

UK brand names: None

Average doses:

- 200-300 mg a day

What form does it come in: Tablet

Does it interact with other medicines: Yes, the following interactions are known:

- The following drugs increase exposure to quinine: cimetidine, phenobarbitol, carbamazepine.
- The following drugs decrease exposure to quinine: rifampicin.
- Quinine increases the concentration or effects of the following drugs: digoxin, amantadine, anticoagulants.
- Quinine decreases the concentration of the following drugs: ciclosporin.
- The following drugs are likely to increase adverse effects with quinine: antiepileptics, moxifloxacin, terfenadine, pimozide, thioridazine, hypoglycaemics, suxamethonium, drugs that prolong QT interval (including amiodarone, moxifloxacin, pimozide, thioridazine and halofantrine).

Drug group: Muscle relaxants – centrally acting

Drug name: Baclofen

UK brand names: Lioresal, Gablofen, Lyflex

Average doses:

- 5-20 mg 3 times a day

What form does it come in: Tablet, solution for injection, solution for infusion, oral solution

Does it interact with other medicines: Yes, the following interactions are known:

- Increased adverse effects may be seen with the following drugs: levodopa, anti-hypertensives, CNS depressants.

Drug name: Tizanidine

UK brand names: None

Average doses:

- 24 mg per day in divided doses (maximum 36 mg)

(Continued)

What form does it come in: Tablet

Does it interact with other medicines: Yes, the following interactions are known:

- The following drugs increase exposure to tizanidine: fluvoxamine, ciprofloxacin, amiodarone, mexiletine, propafenone, verapamil, cimetidine, famotidine, some fluoroquinolones (enoxacin, pefloxacin, norfloxacin), rofecoxib, acyclovir, ticlopidine.
- The following drugs decrease exposure to tizanidine: rifampicin, smoking.
- Increased adverse effects may be seen with the following drugs: drugs prolonging QT interval, anti-hypertensives, including diuretics, beta blockers, digoxin, other CNS depressants.

Drug group: Muscle relaxants – direct acting

Drug name: Dantrolene

UK brand names: Dantrium

Average doses:

- 75-100 mg, 3-4 times per day

What form does it come in: Powder for solution for injection, capsule

Does it interact with other medicines: Yes, the following interactions are known:

- Increased risk of hyperkalaemia and circulatory collapse with diltiazem or verapamil.

DRUG GROUPS/CONCEPT: DRUGS TO TREAT OSTEOPOROSIS

Drugs that treat osteoporosis either reduce bone reabsorption or increase bone formation. Oestrogens play an important role in maintaining bone density in women by increasing osteoblast proliferation and reducing cell death, as well as inhibiting cytokines that recruit osteoclast, causing a reduction in bone reabsorption. The reduction of oestrogens post-menopause increases the risk of osteoporosis. Hormone replacement therapy can help with this, although these treatments are not discussed in this book.

GO FURTHER

Further information on HRT can be found at: https://cks.nice.org.uk/topics/menopause/prescribing-information/hormone-replacement-therapy-hrt/

Bisphonates reduce bone formation by reducing the action of osteoclasts. The bisphosphonates included in this guide prevent the osteoclasts from attaching to bone and therefore they cannot reabsorb bone (Ritter et al., 2020). Oral bisphosphonates are poorly absorbed and have to be taken on an empty stomach but can cause severe oesophageal irritation, and therefore the patient must sit upright or stand and drink plenty of water to prevent oesophageal reflux.

Denosumab is a monoclonal antibody which binds to RANKL. This inhibits the formation, function and survival of osteoclasts, thus reducing bone reabsorption. Strontium also affects the function of osteoclasts and increases apoptosis.

Cholecalciferol (vitamin D3) increases the absorption of calcium and stimulates the synthesis of osteocalcin which is the protein which binds calcium in bones.

Romosozumab is another monoclonal antibody, this time binding to sclerostin. The inactivity of this protein increases the number of osteoblasts and reduces osteoclasts, increasing bone formation and reducing reabsorption.

Teriparatide is a parathyroid hormone treatment which increases the number and activity of osteoblasts.

Drug group: Bisphosphonates

Drug name: Alendronic acid (Alendronate)

UK brand names: Fosamax

Average doses:

- 10 mg per day

What form does it come in: Oral solution, effervescent tablet, tablet

Does it interact with other medicines: Yes, the following interactions are known:

- The following drugs decrease the absorption of alendronate: oral antacids, oral calcium salts, oral magnesium, oral zinc.
- The following drugs increase the risk of unwanted side effects with alendronate (including hypocalcaemia or gastrointestinal bleeding): aminoglycosides, aspirin, NSAIDs, deferasirox.
- Alendronate reduces the effects of parathyroid hormone.

(Continued)

Drug name: Alendronic acid with colecalciferol

UK brand names: Bentexo, Fosavance

Average doses:

- 1 tablet once weekly

What form does it come in: Tablet

Does it interact with other medicines: Yes, the following interactions are known:

- As alendronate.
- The following drugs decrease the effects or exposure to cholecalciferol: antifungals, antiepileptics.
- The following drugs increase risks of unwanted side effects/toxicity with cholecalciferol: digoxin, thiazide diuretics.

Drug name: Ibandronic acid

UK brand names: Bonviva, Bondronat, Iasibon, Quodixor

Average doses:

- Orally 150 mg once a month; by intravenous infusion 3 mg every three months

What form does it come in: Solution for injection, solution for infusion, tablet

Does it interact with other medicines: Yes, the following interactions are known:

- As alendronate.

Drug name: Risedronate sodium

UK brand names: Actonel

Average doses:

- 5 mg per day in women, or 35 mg weekly for males/females

What form does it come in: Tablet

Does it interact with other medicines: Yes, the following interactions are known:

- The following drugs decrease the absorption of risedronate: oral antacids, oral calcium salts, oral magnesium, oral zinc, oral iron.
- The following drugs increase risks of unwanted side effects with alendronate (including hypocalcaemia or gastrointestinal bleeding): aminoglycosides, deferasirox.
- Risedronate reduces the effects of parathyroid hormone.

Drug name: Risedronate with calcium carbonate and cholecalciferol

UK brand names: Actonel Combi

Average doses:

- 1 tablet weekly followed by 1 sachet of granules on days 2-6 of the weekly cycle

What form does it come in: Tablet/granules

Does it interact with other medicines: Yes, the following interactions are known:

- As risedronate.
- The following drugs decrease the effects or exposure to cholecalciferol: antifungals, antiepileptics.
- The following drugs increase risks of unwanted side effects/toxicity with cholecalciferol: digoxin, thiazide diuretic.
- Calcium carbonate reduces the absorption/exposure to the following drugs: acalbrutinib, estramustine, antimalarials, bisphosphonates, dolutegravir, eltrombag, oral iron, hydroxychloroquine, ledipasvir, neratinib, ripivirinem ciproxin, raltegravir, strontium, tetracyclines, levothyroxine, velpatasvir, zinc.
- Ceftriaxone increases the risk of cardiorespiratory arrest when given with calcium carbonate.

Drug name: Zoledronic acid

UK brand names: Aclasta, Zometa

Average doses:

- 5 mg once yearly to every 18 months

What form does it come in: Infusion, solution for infusion

(Continued)

Does it interact with other medicines: Yes, the following interactions are known:

- The following drugs increase risks of unwanted side effects with zoledronate: aminoglycosides.
- Caution with reduced renal function.

Drug group: Calcium regulating drugs -bone reabsorption inhibitors

Drug name: Strontium ranelate

UK brand names: None

Average doses:

- 2 g per day

What form does it come in: Granules

Does it interact with other medicines: Yes, the following interactions are known:

- The following drugs increase the absorption of / exposure to strontium: oral antacids, oral calcium salts.
- Strontium reduces the absorption of the following drugs: quinolones, tetracyclines.
- Strontium increases the risk of thromboembolism with other drugs that also increase the risk, for example: methotrexate, tamoxifen, tranexamic acid.

Drug group: Calcium regulating drugs - parathyroid hormones and analogues

Drug name: Teriparatide

UK brand names: Forsteo, Movymia, Terrosa

Average doses:

- 20 micrograms per day for up to 24 months

What form does it come in: Solution for injection

Does it interact with other medicines: Yes, the following interactions are known:

- Caution when given with digoxin, may increase likelihood of digoxin toxicity due to transient hypercalcaemia.

Drug group: Drugs affecting bone structure and metabolism - monoclonal antibodies

Drug name: Denosumab

UK brand names: Prolia

Average doses:

- 60 mg every six months

What form does it come in: Solution for injection

Does it interact with other medicines: No

Drug name: Romosozumab

UK brand names: Evenity

Average doses:

- 210 mg once a month for 12 months

What form does it come in: Solution for injection

Does it interact with other medicines: No

DRUG GROUPS/CONCEPT: DRUGS TO TREAT MACULAR DEGENERATION

Drugs treatments for wet macular degeneration aim to reduce the formation of new blood vessels under and around the macula. Vascular endothelial growth factor inhibitor reduces the production of growth factors that stimulate the production of blood vessels. Photosensitisers cause vascular occlusion and damage or death of the endothelial cells of the new blood vessels (Datapharm, 2023). Vitamin supplements are sometimes suggested to slow dry macular degeneration along with a healthy lifestyle.

Drug group: Vascular endothelial growth factor inhibitors

Drug name: Aflibercept

UK brand names: Eylea

Average doses:

- 2 mg every month or two-monthly

What form does it come in: Solution for injection

Does it interact with other medicines: No

Drug name: Brolucizamab

UK brand names: Beovu

Average doses:

- 6 mg once a month

What form does it come in: Solution for injection

Does it interact with other medicines: No

Drug name: Ranibizumab

UK brand names: Lucentis

Average doses:

- 500 micrograms once a month

What form does it come in: Solution for injection

Does it interact with other medicines: Yes, the following interactions are known:

- Increased risk of bleeding events when given with the following drugs: coumarins, danaparoid, heparin, low-molecular weight heparins, phenindione, thrombin inhibitors.

Drug group: Photosensitisers

Drug name: Verteporfin

UK brand names: Visudyne

Average doses:

- 6 mg/m^2 (dosed by body surface area)

What form does it come in: Powder for solution for infusion

Does it interact with other medicines: Yes, the following interactions are known:

- Caution when administering with other photosensitising drugs.

DRUG GROUPS/CONCEPT: DRUGS TO TREAT GLAUCOMA

The treatment of glaucoma aims to reduce intraocular pressure by either reducing the production of aqueous humour or increasing its outflow. Beta adrenoceptor antagonists, alpha adrenoceptor agonists and carbonic anhydrase inhibitors all reduce the production of aqueous humour in the ciliary body of the eye. Parasympathomimetics cause contraction of the smooth muscle of the ciliary body, widening the outflow at the trabecular meshwork and canal of Schlemm (Schmidl et al., 2015). Prostaglandins and prostamines increase outflow of aqueous humour through an alternative pathway where the fluid moves through the ciliary muscle and body into the choroid and sclera. Eye drops are used to treat glaucoma which reduces but does not eliminate systemic side effects.

Drug group: Beta adrenoceptor antagonists

Drug name: Betaxolol

UK brand names: Betoptic

Average doses:

- Apply twice daily

What form does it come in: Eye drops

Does it interact with other medicines: Yes, the following interactions are known:

- The following drugs increase risks of unwanted side effects when given with betaxolol: aminophylline, propafenone, mefloquine, diltiazem, verapamil, ergometrine, ergotamine, lanreotide, mexiletine, dobutamine, adrenaline, noradrenaline, theophylline.

Drug name: Levobunolol hydroxide

UK brand names: Betagan

Average doses:

- Apply 1-2 times daily

What form does it come in: Eye drops

Does it interact with other medicines: Yes, the following interactions are known:

- The following drugs increase risks of unwanted side effects when given with levobunolol: aminophylline, propafenone, mefloquine, diltiazem, verapamil, ergometrine, ergotamine, lanreotide, mexiletine, dobutamine, adrenaline, noradrenaline, theophylline.

Drug name: Timolol maleate

UK brand names: Eysano, Timoptol, Tiopex

Average doses:

- Apply 1-2 times daily

What form does it come in: Eye drops, eye gel

Does it interact with other medicines: Yes, the following interactions are known:

- The following drugs increase exposure to timolol: propafenone.
- The following drugs increase risks of unwanted side effects when given with timolol: aminophylline, propafenone, mefloquine, diltiazem, verapamil, ergometrine, ergotamine, lanreotide, mexiletine, dobutamine, adrenaline, noradrenaline, theophylline.

Drug group: Carbonic anhydrase inhibitors

Drug name: Acetazolamide

UK brand names: Diamox, Eytazox

Average doses:

- Oral: 0.25–1 g per day in divided doses

What form does it come in: Tablet, powder for solution for injection, modified release capsule

Does it interact with other medicines: Yes, the following interactions are known:

- The following drugs increase risks of unwanted side effects when given with acetazolamide: valporate, zonisamide, aspirin.
- Acetazolamide alters the concentration of lithium.
- Acetazolamide decreases the efficiency of methenamine.
- Acetazolamide increases the urinary excretion of methotrexate.

Drug name: Brinzolamide

UK brand names: Azopt

Average doses:

- Apply 2–3 times daily

What form does it come in: Eye drops

Does it interact with other medicines: No

(Continued)

Drug name: Brinzolamide with brimonidine

UK brand names: Simbrinza

Average doses:

- Apply 1 drop twice a day

What form does it come in: Eye drops

Does it interact with other medicines: Yes, the following interactions are known:

- Tricyclic antidepressants blunt the effects of brinzolamide with brimonidine.
- The following drugs increase risks of unwanted side effects when administered along with brinzolamide with brimonidine: anti-hypertensives, cardiac glycosides, oral carbonic anhydrase inhibitors.

Drug name: Brinzolamide with timolol

UK brand names: Azarga

Average doses:

- Apply twice a day

What form does it come in: eye drops

Does it interact with other medicines: Yes, the following interactions are known:

- As timolol.

Drug name: Dorzolamide

UK brand names: Eydelto, Trusopt

Average doses:

- Apply 2–3 times a day

What form does it come in: Eye drops

Does it interact with other medicines: No

Drug name: Dorzolamide with timolol

UK brand names: Cosopt, Eylamdo

Average doses:

- Apply twice a day

What form does it come in: Eye drops

Does it interact with other medicines: Yes, the following interactions are known:

- As timolol.

Drug group: Miotics - parasympathomimetics

Drug name: Pilocarpine

UK brand names: None

Average doses:

- Apply four times per day

What form does it come in: Eye drops

Does it interact with other medicines: No

Drug group: Prostaglandins and analogues

Drug name: Latanoprost

UK brand names: Medizol, Monopost, Xalatan

Average doses:

- Apply once daily

What form does it come in: Eye drops

Does it interact with other medicines: No

(Continued)

Drug name: Latanoprost with timolol

UK brand names: Fixapost, Medox, Xalacom

Average doses:

- Apply once daily

What form does it come in: Eye drops

Does it interact with other medicines: Yes, the following interactions are known:

- As timolol.

Drug name: Tafluprost

UK brand names: Saflutan

Average doses:

- Apply once daily

What form does it come in: Eye drops

Does it interact with other medicines: No

Drug name: Tafluprost with timolol

UK brand names: Taptiqom

Average doses:

- Apply 1 drop daily

What form does it come in: Eye drops

Does it interact with other medicines: Yes, the following interactions are known:

- As timolol.

Drug name: Travoprost

UK brand names: Bondulc, Travatan

Average doses:

- Apply once daily

What form does it come in: Eye drops

Does it interact with other medicines: No

Drug name: Travoprost with timolol

UK brand names: Duotrav

Average doses:

- Apply once daily

What form does it come in: Eye drops

Does it interact with other medicines: Yes, the following interactions are known:

- As timolol.

Drug group: Prostamides

Drug name: Bimatoprost

UK brand names: Eyeida, Lumigan

Average doses:

- Apply once daily

What form does it come in: Eye drops

Does it interact with other medicines: No

(Continued)

Drug name: Bimatoprost with timolol

UK brand names: Eyzeetan, Ganfort

Average doses:

- Apply once daily

What form does it come in: Eye drops

Does it interact with other medicines: Yes, the following interactions are known:

- As timolol.

Drug group: Alpha 2 - adrenoceptor agonists

Drug name: Apraclonidine

UK brand names: Iopidine

Average doses:

- Before/after surgery: 1 drop an hour before surgery and 1 drop immediately after. For short-term treatment 1 drop three times per day for up to a month

What form does it come in: eye drops

Does it interact with other medicines: Yes, the following interactions are known:

- The following drugs decrease the effect of apraclonidine: amphetamines, methylphenidate, sympathomimetics (inotrope, vasoconstrictor).

Drug name: Brimonidine tartrate

UK brand names: Alphagan, Brymont

Average doses:

- Apply twice daily

What form does it come in: Eye drops

Does it interact with other medicines: Yes, the following interactions are known:

- Tricyclic antidepressants blunt the effects of brimonidine.
- The following drugs increase risks of unwanted side effects when administered along with brimonidine: anti-hypertensives, cardiac glycosides, oral carbonic anhydrase inhibitors.

Drug name: Brimonidine with timolol

UK brand names: Combigan

Average doses:

- Apply twice daily

What form does it come in: Eye drops

Does it interact with other medicines: Yes, the following interactions are known:

- As timolol.
- As brimonidine.

DRUGS FOR DEGENERATIVE CONDITIONS IN PREGNANCY AND BREASTFEEDING

As some degenerative conditions are more prevalent in older people, pregnancy and breast-feeding may not be a consideration, however as diagnosis improves and conditions are recognised earlier this may change. Many of the degenerative conditions are complex and would require a multidisciplinary approach to treatment during pregnancy and postpartum.

There is some evidence that during pregnancy, symptoms of multiple sclerosis reduce, and that remission is more common, however the opposite may be true postpartum. Several treatments for multiple sclerosis are given infrequently and timings may be adjusted around pregnancy. Effective contraception is advised if taking teriflunomide during treatment and for two years after and for two to three months after for fingolimod, ozanimod and siponimod (Joint Formulary Committee, 2024).

There are few reported cases of people with Parkinson's disease becoming pregnant but limited evidence seems to suggest that levodopa and cabidopa or benerazide may be relatively safe during pregnancy (Olivola et al., 2020), although they may suppress lactation and are found in breast milk. Amantadine should be avoided in pregnancy and breastfeeding due to toxicity and potential teratogenic affects (Joint Formulary Committee, 2024).

Bisphosphonates have a terminal half-life of up to ten years as they are stored in bones and therefore foetal exposure can occur long after treatment, however there is limited evidence about risks in pregnancy (UK Teratology Information Service, 2023). It is advised that contraception is taken during and for five months after treatment with denosumab (Joint Formulary Committee, 2024).

Whilst eye drops might seem to be safe, systemic absorption needs to be considered, for example timolol can cause bradycardia in the foetus and newborn (UK Teratology Information Service, 2023).

LEARNING FROM A CASE STUDY: TEST YOUR KNOWLEDGE

Arthur is a 72-year-old man who is seeing his doctor for a review following a fall. He lives in a residential home with support from carers. He was diagnosed with Parkinson's disease ten years ago and also has open angle glaucoma. On presentation he has a shuffling gait, muscle stiffness and a tremor. He is reporting that his symptoms have become worse over the last six months, and it is particularly difficult as he must rely on carers to help him with his medication. He is also feeling depressed and isolated. He is currently prescribed co-beneldopa 200 mg four times a day and timolol eye drops twice a day.

1   Why might Arthur's medication not be as effective as it was?
2   What advice would you give Arthur and his carers about administration of his medication?
3   What other medication or treatment might be appropriate for Arthur's increasing symptoms?
4   Would social prescribing be appropriate in this case and if so what would you suggest?

IF I REMEMBER 5 THINGS FROM THIS CHAPTER:

1   The causes of degenerative diseases are often multifactorial.
2   Degenerative diseases increase with age and may co-occur.
3   Interactions need to be considered even with eye drops due to systemic absorption.
4   Symptom control rather than cure is often the aim in the treatment of degenerative conditions.
5   Social prescribing may be beneficial.

ANSWERS TO CASE STUDY QUESTIONS

1   Arthur has had Parkinson's disease for at least ten years and as the disease progresses, so the number of dopaminergic cells in the substantia nigra reduces. Co-beneldopa can only work if there are cells for the dopamine to bind to and therefore as the disease progresses, this treatment becomes less effective.

2   Arthur is relying on the carers to help him with his medication. It may be that he is unable to open the bottles or have the dexterity to administer eye drops in particular. Co-beneldopa need to be administered at regular intervals as there is a tendency to a stop-start action. Arthur will have increased levels of rigidity and difficulty initiating movements if too much time passes between his medication doses, and he will have particular difficulty first thing in the morning until the medication takes effect. The need for timely help with medications should be reiterated.

3   Arthur should be reviewed by his neurologist and additional drugs may be added to his regimen. These may include COMT inhibitors, MOA-B inhibitors, antimuscarinics or dopaminergic drugs. Arthur may also benefit from a psychiatric consultation and possibly antidepressants. Arthur may benefit from a deep brain stimulator and this should also be discussed.

4   Arthur is feeling isolated and would benefit from social prescribing. He may wish to take part in a group to talk with others who have Parkinson's disease. Finding out about his hobbies and interests would help to identify what he would enjoy doing. Physical exercise can help with muscle strength and endurance as well as improving other disease symptoms and general health and wellbeing. Singing has also been shown to be beneficial.

REFERENCES AND RECOMMENDED READING

Chang, C. and Ramphul, K. (2022) *Amantadine*. Treasure Island, FL: StatPearls Publishing. Available at: www.ncbi.nlm.nih.gov/books/NBK499953/

Datapharm (2023) *Electronic Medicines Compendium*. Available at: www.medicines.org.uk/emc

International Osteoporosis Foundation and Scope 21 (2021) Epidemiology, burden, and treatment of osteoporosis in the United Kingdom. Available at: www.osteoporosis. foundation/sites/iofbonehealth/files/scope-2021/UK%20report.pdf

Joint Formulary Committee (2024) British National Formulary. Available at: https://bnf. nice.org.uk/

National Institute for Health and Care Excellence (NICE) (2019) Motor neurone disease: assessment and management NICE guideline [NG42] Available at: https://www.nice.org. uk/guidance/ng42/chapter/recommendations#managing-symptoms

National Institute for Health and Care Excellence (NICE) (2022a) Glaucoma. Available at: https://cks.nice.org.uk/topics/glaucoma/

National Institute for Health and Care Excellence (NICE) (2022b) Multiple sclerosis in adults: Management. Nice guideline [NG220]. Available at: www.nice.org.uk/guidance/ng220

Olivola, S., Xodo, S., Olivola, E., Cecchini, F., Londero, A. P., & Driul, L. (2020). Parkinson's Disease in Pregnancy: A Case Report and Review of the Literature. *Frontiers in Neurology*, 10, 1349–1349. https://doi.org/10.3389/fneur.2019.01349

Parkinson's UK (2022) Written evidence submitted by Parkinson's UK (RTR0067). Available at: https://committees.parliament.uk/writtenevidence/42721/pdf/#:~:text=About%20 Parkinson's,-4.&text=Currently%20145%2C000%20people%20in%20the,fifth%20to%20 172%2C000%20by%202030

Public Health England (2020) Multiple sclerosis: prevalence, incidence and smoking status – data briefing. Available at: www.gov.uk/government/publications/multiple-sclerosis-prevalence-incidence-and-smoking-status/multiple-sclerosis-prevalence-incidence-and-smoking-status-data-briefing

Ritter, J.M., Flower, R., Henderson, H., Kong Loke, Y., MacEwan, D. and Rang, H.P. (2020) *Rang and Dale's Pharmacology* (9th edn). Edinburgh: Elsevier.

Schmidl, D., Schmetterer, L., Garhöfer, G. and Popa-Cherecheanu, A. (2015) Pharmacotherapy of glaucoma. *Journal of Ocular Pharmacology and Therapeutics: The Official Journal of the Association for Ocular Pharmacology and Therapeutics*, 31(2), 63–77. https://doi.org/10.1089/jop.2014.0067

UK Teratology Information Service (2023) UKTIS monographs. Available at: https://uktis.org/mongraphs

Wei, W., Ma, D., Li, L. and Zhang, L. (2021) Progress in the application of drugs for the treatment of multiple sclerosis. *Frontiers in Pharmacology*, 12. https://doi.org/10.3389/fphar.2021.724718

Willihnganz, M.J., Gurevitz, S.L. and Clayton, B.D. (2020) *Clayton's Basic Pharmacology for Nurses*. St Louis: Elsevier.

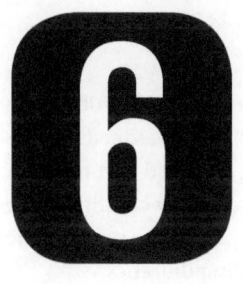

6 MEDICINES FOR CIRCULATORY AND TRANSPORTATION CONDITIONS

RACHAEL MAJOR

AFTER READING THIS CHAPTER YOU WILL BE ABLE TO:

- Consider the impact of cardiovascular disease on UK society and healthcare.
- Discuss the role that the renin angiotensin aldosterone system has on regulation of blood pressure and drugs that act within this system.
- Outline the common drugs used to treat cardiovascular disorders and their actions and interactions.
- Apply knowledge around medications for cardiovascular disorders to support holistic clinical decision making.

OVERVIEW

Cardiovascular disease is the second most common cause of avoidable mortality behind cancers in all countries of the UK (Office for National Statistics, 2022) and heart and circulatory conditions are costing the NHS in England at least £7.4 million a year as one in four people are living with cardiac and circulatory conditions (Haque, 2020). The number of prescriptions written for the cardiovascular system rose by 36% in the ten years from 2006 to 2016, with the majority of that increase being attributed to lipid lowering drugs (statins) and drugs to treat hypertension (Palmer, 2020).

Hypertension affects one in four people in England and the rates are rising across the world. It is the single largest risk factor for heart failure, coronary artery disease, renal failure and stroke (Gov.uk, 2017). In many cases, dietary and lifestyle factors also need to be considered alongside medications. Increased exercise, weight loss, dietary modifications and smoking cessation can greatly reduce morbidity and risk factors.

This chapter will explore drugs that treat common cardiac and circulatory disorders such as heart failure, cardiac arrythmias, hypercholesterolaemia and angina, as well as medications affecting haemostasis such as antiplatelets and anticoagulants. It must be noted that many of the drugs addressed in this chapter are used to treat more than one circulatory condition due to common causes, comorbidities and drugs acting on more than one part of the system. The chapter will start by addressing drugs that affect blood pressure including diuretics.

GO FURTHER

The British Heart Foundation has a wide range of information for both healthcare professionals and patients on cardiovascular disease, lifestyle modification and treatments which is available at www.bhf.org.uk/

The medicines list
- Angiotensin converting enzyme (ACE) inhibitors
- Angiotensin II inhibitors
- Renin inhibitors
- Calcium channel antagonists
- β adrenergic receptor antagonists (β blockers)
- α adrenergic receptor antagonist (α blockers)
- Nitrates
- Diuretics
- Class I antiarrhythmics
- Class III antiarrhythmics
- Adenosine
- Cardiac glycosides
- Lipid modifying drugs
- Antiplatelet drugs
- Antithrombin drugs
- Fibrinolytics

DRUG CONCEPT: DRUGS AFFECTING BLOOD PRESSURE AND DRUGS FOR HEART FAILURE

When discussing hypertension, it is important to understand the renin, angiotensin, aldosterone system (RAAS). Renin is released from the kidneys in response to raised blood pressure. Renin converts angiotensinogen (which is mainly released from the liver) to angiotensin I. Angiotensin I is converted to angiotensin II by angiotensin converting enzyme (ACE), which is predominantly released from the lungs. Angiotensin II causes vasoconstriction increasing peripheral resistance and in turn blood pressure. Angiotensin II also has a direct effect on the proximal convoluted tubule in the kidney, increasing sodium reabsorption which causes water to be pulled into the blood through osmosis and increases blood pressure. Angiotensin II has a direct effect on the brain, stimulating the thirst centre in the hypothalamus, and reducing the sensitivity of the baroreceptor reflex to hypertension, potentially leading to chronic hypertension. Angiotensin II also causes the release of aldosterone from the adrenal cortex and antidiuretic hormone (ADH or vasopressin) from the pituitary gland. Aldosterone acts on the distal convoluted tubules and collecting ducts in the kidney to increase the reabsorption of sodium and water, thus increasing blood volume and therefore blood pressure. ADH acts to constrict vascular smooth muscle which causes an increase in peripheral resistance. ADH also acts on the collecting duct of the kidney tubule to increase reabsorption of water, increasing blood volume; both mechanisms will increase blood pressure.

ACE inhibitors act to inhibit the conversion of angiotensin I to angiotensin II, preventing vasoconstriction and decreasing vascular resistance as well as reducing aldosterone production. ACE also acts to inhibit bradykinin, an inflammatory mediator which dilates blood vessels, thus inhibiting this effect can also decrease peripheral resistance and reduce blood pressure. ACE inhibitors are also used in heart failure by reducing vasoconstriction which is initiated by reduced cardiac output. This reduces the strain on the heart, which increases life expectancy and hospital admissions (Ashelford et al., 2019).

Angiotensin II receptor blockers (ARBs) block the angiotensin receptors and therefore the effects of angiotensin II. As the effects of the RAAS system diminish with age ACE inhibitors are not first line treatment in the over 55 age group but they are still very effective and should be offered to all patients with hypertension and type 2 diabetes (NICE, 2022). Both ACE inhibitors and ARBs have been found to be less effective in patients with a Black African or Afro-Caribbean family origin.

There is one renin inhibitor currently licensed, aliskiren, although not commonly used due to increased side effects and being contraindicated in those with renal impairment or diabetes (Miller and Arnold, 2022). Renin inhibitors block the effects of renin and therefore the production of angiotensin I.

Calcium channel blockers (CCBs) are one of the first line treatments for hypertension in the over 55-year-old age group without type 2 diabetes or those of any age without diabetes with a Black African or Afro-Caribbean family origin. CCBs block the entry of calcium into cells via calcium channels and can act on both cardiac and smooth muscle. Different types of CCBs have variable effects on cardiac or smooth muscle, for example verapamil preferentially affects cardiac muscle, whereas the dihydropyridines (e.g. nifedipine and amlodipine) have more effect on smooth muscle, and diltiazem affects both. In relation to blood pressure, CCBs cause vasodilation of arteries and arterioles and thus reduce peripheral resistance and reduce blood pressure. They also cause coronary artery vasodilatation and are therefore used in variant angina when the arteries spasm. Verapamil acts to slow conduction in the sinoatrial and atrioventricular (AV) nodes of the heart and is therefore used in supraventricular tachycardia (SVT) (now more often adenosine). However, it can cause AV block and bradycardia.

Beta-adrenergic receptor antagonists (β-blockers) have several actions, including reducing blood pressure. These drugs block the action of adrenaline and noradrenaline produced by the sympathetic nervous system which is most active during stress and exercise. Selective β-blockers act on β1 receptors in the heart, whereas less selective drugs such as propranolol also act on the β2 receptors found in the airways and can cause severe bronchospasm in patients with asthma which will not respond to salbutamol, other β2 agonists or adrenaline. β-blockers reduce blood pressure by reducing cardiac output, by reducing force and rate of contraction of the heart muscle, reducing the release of renin and in general reducing the activity of the sympathetic nervous system (Ritter et al., 2020). β-blockers reduce the workload of the heart and therefore the metabolic requirements of the heart and are therefore used as a treatment following myocardial infarction and in heart failure (NICE, 2018). They also increase the refractory period of the atrioventricular node and therefore are used to reduce the risk of SVT.

Alpha-adrenoceptor antagonists, in particular selective α1 adrenoceptor antagonists, act on smooth muscle to cause vasodilation and therefore reduce blood pressure. There are also drugs that have both selective α1 and β1 blocker activity and therefore reduce heart rate and force of contraction and vasodilation of arterial smooth muscle (Ritter et al., 2020).

Nitrates are potent vasodilators used to treat angina and in myocardial infarction. They are a source of nitric oxide which causes epithelial and vascular smooth muscle to relax, increasing blood flow to the affected area of the heart.

Diuretics are another major group of drugs that are used to treat hypertension and also heart failure. Thiazide diuretics and related drugs act on the distal convoluted tubule in the nephron of the kidney to block the reabsorption of sodium. Water follows sodium causing an increase in diuresis and therefore a reduction in blood volume. They also cause vasodilation, increasing their anti-hypertensive effects. Thiazide like diuretics are also recommended for treatment of hypertension with evidence of heart failure (NICE, 2022). Loop diuretics act on the Loop of Henle in the kidney tubule. They are strong diuretics causing the loss of sodium, potassium and chloride, along with water, into the urine, as well as having a vasodilatory effect. They are used to treat pulmonary oedema and peripheral oedema, secondary to heart failure. Aldosterone antagonists act on the distal convoluted tubule. They cause the reabsorption of potassium instead of sodium and are therefore 'potassium sparing'. Other potassium-sparing diuretics are amiloride and triamterene, which block the reabsorption of sodium in the collecting duct and therefore preserve potassium (which is normally exchanged for sodium). Potassium-sparing diuretics may be combined with loop or thiazide diuretics to increase diuresis, whilst improving electrolyte balance (Ritter et al., 2020).

Low blood pressure can also be a problem due to reduced perfusion to essential organs. Sympathomimetics mirror the action of the sympathetic nervous system, increasing rate and force of contraction of the heart and causing vasoconstriction of peripheries, thus increasing cardiac output and peripheral resistance and therefore blood pressure. Sympathomimetic inotropes such as dobutamine also act to increase the force of contraction of the heart by acting on the β2 adrenergic receptors. These drugs are administered in emergency and critical care settings and will not be discussed in this book.

Drug group: Angiotensin converting enzyme inhibitors

Drug name: Captopril

UK brand names: Noyada

Average doses:

- 6.25-25 mg initially twice a day then increase to 150 mg daily in 2 divided doses (once daily may be appropriate if on other anti-hypertensives)

What form does it come in: Tablets, oral solution

Does it interact with other medicines: Yes, the following interactions are known:

- Increased risk of side effects, reactions of renal impairment when administered with the following: aliskiren, allopurinol, azathioprine, everolimus, gold, temsirolimus.
- Administration with icatibant reduced the efficacy of both drugs.
- ACE inhibitors increase the concentration of lithium.

Drug name: Fosinopril sodium

UK brand names: None

Average doses:

- 10 mg initially for four weeks then increase up to 40 mg per day

What form does it come in: Tablets

Does it interact with other medicines: Yes, the following interactions are known:

- As captopril.

Drug name: Imidapril

UK brand names: Tanatril

Average doses:

- Initially 2.5-5 mg, increase slowly to 10 mg per day, 20 mg per day maximum dose

(Continued)

What form does it come in: Tablets

Does it interact with other medicines: Yes, the following interactions are known:

- As captopril.

Drug name: Lisinopril

UK brand names: Zestril

Average doses:

- 2.5-10 mg initially depending on condition being treated. Maintenance dose usually 10-20 mg. Maximum dose 80 mg per day

What form does it come in: Tablet, oral solution

Does it interact with other medicines: Yes, the following interactions are known:

- As captopril.

Drug name: Perindopril arginine

UK brand names: Coversyl Arginine

Average doses:

- Initially 2.5-5 mg then increase to 5-10 mg per day

What form does it come in: Tablet

Does it interact with other medicines: Yes, the following interactions are known:

- As captopril.

Drug name: Quinapril

UK brand names: Accupro

Average doses:

- Initially 2.5 or 10 mg, maintenance dose 20-40 mg per day, maximum dose 80 mg

What form does it come in: Tablet

Does it interact with other medicines: Yes, the following interactions are known:

- As captopril.
- Quinapril decreases absorption of oral tetracyclines.

Drug name: Ramipril

UK brand names: None

Average doses:

- Initially 1.25-2.5 mg per day, increase to 5-10 mg per day

What form does it come in: Tablet, capsule, oral solution

Does it interact with other medicines: Yes, the following interactions are known:

- As captopril.

Drug name: Trandolapril

UK brand names: None

Average doses:

- Initially 500 micrograms daily increase slowly to 1-2 mg daily maximum dose 4 mg per day

What form does it come in: Capsule

Does it interact with other medicines: Yes, the following interactions are known:

- As captopril.

Drug group: Angiotensin II receptor antagonists

Drug name: Azilsartan medoxonil

UK brand names: Edarbi

Average doses:

- 20-40 mg initially, increase slowly up to 80 mg maximum per day

What form does it come in: Tablet

Does it interact with other medicines: Yes, the following interactions are known:

- Increased risk of renal impairment when administered with aliskiren.
- Increases exposure to lithium.

Drug name: Candesartan cilexetil

UK brand names: None

Average doses:

- 4-8 mg initially, increase slowly up to 32 mg maximum dose per day

What form does it come in: Tablet

Does it interact with other medicines: Yes, the following interactions are known:

- As azilsartan.

Drug name: Eprosartan

UK brand names: Teveten

Average doses:

- 600 mg per day

What form does it come in: Tablet

Does it interact with other medicines: Yes, the following interactions are known:

- As azilsartan.

Drug name: Irbesartan

UK brand names: Aprovel, Ifirmasta

Average doses:

- Initially 75-150 mg daily, increased to 300 mg per day

What form does it come in: Tablet

Does it interact with other medicines: Yes, the following interactions are known:

- As azilsartan.

Drug name: Losartan potassium

UK brand names: Cozaar

Average doses:

- Initially 12.5-50 mg, increase slowly to 100-150 mg per day

What form does it come in: Tablet

Does it interact with other medicines: Yes, the following interactions are known:

- As azilsartan.

Drug name: Olmesartan medoxomil

UK brand names: Olmetec

Average doses:

- Initially 10 mg per day, increase to 20 mg, maximum dose 40 mg per day

What form does it come in: Tablet

Does it interact with other medicines: Yes, the following interactions are known:

- As azilsartan.

(Continued)

Drug name: Telmisartan

UK brand names: Micardis, Tolura

Average doses:

- Initially 20-40 mg per day, increase if required after four weeks up to 80 mg per day

What form does it come in: Tablet

Does it interact with other medicines: Yes, the following interactions are known:

- As azilsartan.

Drug name: Valsartan

UK brand names: None

Average doses:

- Initially 20-80 mg, increase slowly up to 160-320 mg per day if required

What form does it come in: Tablet, capsule

Does it interact with other medicines: Yes, the following interactions are known:

- As azilsartan.
- Filgotinib increases exposure to valsartan.

Drug group: Renin inhibitors

Drug name: Aliskiren

UK brand names: Rasilez

Average doses:

- 150-300 mg per day

What form does it come in: Tablet

Does it interact with other medicines: Yes, the following interactions are known:

- The following drugs reduce levels of alskiren: carbamazepine, pitolisant, rifamycins, St John's Wort, apple, orange, and grapefruit juice.
- The following drugs reduce levels of alskiren: amiodarone, dronedarone, antifungals (azoles), verapamil, ceritinib, ciclosporin, eliglustat, HIV-protease inhibitors, lapatinib, macrolides (azithromycin, clarithromycin, erythromycin), mirabegron, paritaprevir, mirabegron, paritaprevir, ranolazine, statins, velpatasvir, vemurafenib.
- ACE inhibitors and angiotensin II receptor antagonists increase the risk of renal impairment if given with alskiren.
- Alskiren reduced exposure to loop diuretics.

Drug group: Calcium channel antagonists (dihydropyridine)

Drug name: Amlodipine

UK brand names: Istin

Average doses:

- 5–10 mg per day

What form does it come in: Oral solution, tablet

Does it interact with other medicines: Yes, the following interactions are known:

- The following drugs increase exposure to amlodipine: dronedarone, antiepileptics, mitotane, tocilizumab, rifamycins, St John's Wort.
- The following drugs increase exposure to amlodipine: anti-androgens, antifungals (azoles), cobicistat, crizotinib, bosentan, grapefruit juice, grazoprevir, HIV-protease inhibitors, Idelalisib, imatinib, letermovir, macrolides, neurokinin-1 receptor antagonists, nilotinib, diltiazem, verapamil.
- Amlodipine increases exposure to: atorvastatin, lomitapide.
- The following drugs increase adverse effects when given with amlodipine: mefloquine, magnesium, efavirenz, nevirapine, temsirolimus.

(Continued)

Drug name: Nicardipine hydrochloride

UK brand names: Cardene

Average doses:

- Orally: initially 20 mg three times a day, increasing slowly to 60-120 mg per day. By intravenous infusion: initially 3-5 mg/hour increasing to maximum of 15 mg/hour, reduce in renal impairment

What form does it come in: Solution for injection, capsule

Does it interact with other medicines: Yes, the following interactions are known:

- As amlodipine
- As Nicardipine increases the concentration of ciclosporin.

Drug name: Nifedipine

UK brand names: Adanif, Adipine, Fortipine, Nidef, Nifedipres, Tensipine, Valni

Average doses:

- 20-90 mg per day. Note different brands have different dosages

What form does it come in: Modified release tablet, modified release capsule

Does it interact with other medicines: Yes, the following interactions are known:

- As amlodipine

Drug group: Calcium channel antagonists

Drug name: Diltiazem hydrochloride

UK brand names: Retalzem, Tildiem, Adizem, Angitil, Dilcadia, Slozem, Uard, Viazem, Zemret

Average doses:

- 60 mg three times a day increasing to 360 mg per day. Note different brands have different dosages

What form does it come in: Modified release tablet, modified release capsule

Does it interact with other medicines: Yes, there are a large number of interactions known as it is an inhibitor of the drug metabolising enzyme CYP3A4, some of which are included here:

- The following drugs increase exposure to diltiazem: cobicistat, HIV-protease inhibitors, idelalisib, macrolides, aprepitant.
- The following drugs decreases exposure to diltiazem: antiandrogens, antiepileptics, endothelin receptor antagonists, milotane, NNRTIs, monoclonal antibodies, St Johns Wort.
- Diltiazem increases exposure to: antiarrhythmics (dronedarone, amiodarone, propafenone), antiepileptics, antifungals, abemaciclib, aldosterone antagonists, antipsychotics (2nd generation), aprepitant, bedaquiline, benzodiazepines, buspirone, CCBs, ciclosporin, cimetidine, colchicine, corticosteroids, darifenacin, dienogest, digoxin, dopamine receptor agonists, elexacaftor, protein kinase inhibitors, tyrosine kinase inhibitors, fingolimod, guanfacine, ivacaftor, ivabradine, midostaurin, naldemedine, naloxegol, phosphodiesterase type-5 inhibitors, opioids, oxybutynin pimozide, ranolazine sirolimus, SSRIs, statins, saxagliptin, tacrolimus, tamsulosin, taxanes, tezcaftor, tolerodine, tolvaptan, trazodone, ventroclax, vinca alkaloids, zopiclone.
- The following drugs increase adverse effects when given with diltiazem: mefloquine, β-blockers, dantrolene, domperidone, ergometrine, lithium, mexiletine, temsirolimus.

Drug name: Verapamil hydrochloride

UK brand names: Securon, Vera-Til, Verapress, Vertab

Average doses:

- 40–480 mg per day orally. Note different brands have different dosages. 5–10 mg by slow intravenous injection

What form does it come in: Modified release tablet, tablet, solution for injection, oral solution

Does it interact with other medicines: Yes, there are a large number of interactions known as it is an inhibitor of CYP3A4, some of which are included here:

- As diltiazem.
- Verapamil increases exposure to: aliskiren, abixaban, dabigatran, doxorubicin, bictegravir fidaxomicin, panobinostat, pibrentasvir.
- Grapefruit juice increases exposure to verapamil.
- The following drugs increase adverse effects when given with verapamil: flecainide.

Drug group: β-adrenoceptor blockers (non-selective) (beta-blockers)

Drug name: Nadolol

UK brand names: Corgard

Average doses:

- 40-80 mg initially up to 240 mg per day

What form does it come in: Tablet

Does it interact with other medicines: Yes, the following interactions are known:

- The following drugs increase the risk of adverse events with nadolol: aminophylline, class I and class III antiarrhythmics, mefloquine, diltiazem, verapamil, ergometrine, lanreotide, mexiletine, sympathomimetics theophylline.
- The following drugs increase exposure to nadolol: antifungals, ciclosporin HIV-protease inhibitors, lapatinib, macrolides, ranolazine, vemurafenib.

Drug name: Propranolol hydrochloride

UK brand names: Bedranol, Beta-Prograne

Average doses:

- 10-320 mg daily in divided doses per day, dependent on condition

What form does it come in: Oral solution, modified release capsule, tablet

Does it interact with other medicines: Yes, the following interactions are known:

- The following drugs increase the risk of adverse events with propranolol: aminophylline, class I and class III antiarrhythmics, mefloquine, diltiazem, verapamil, ergometrine, lanreotide, mexiletine, sympathomimetics, theophylline.
- The following drugs increase exposure to propranolol: dacomitinib, eliglustat, fluvoxamine, rizatriptan.
- The following drugs reduce exposure to propranolol: antiepileptics, rifamycins.

Drug name: Sotalol hydrochloride

UK brand names: Beta-Cardone, Sotacor

Average doses:

- 80 mg initially increasing to 160–320 mg per day, maximum of 480–640 mg per day

What form does it come in: Tablet

Does it interact with other medicines: Yes, the following interactions are known:

- The following drugs increase the risk of adverse events with sotalol: aminophylline, class I and class III antiarrhythmics, chloroprocaine, mefloquine, diltiazem, verapamil, ergometrine, lanreotide, mexiletine, sympathomimetics, theophylline.

Drug name: Timolol maleate

UK brand names: None

Average doses:

- 10 mg initially, up to 60 mg per day maximum dose

What form does it come in: Tablet

Does it interact with other medicines: Yes, the following interactions are known:

- The following drugs increase the risk of adverse events with timolol: aminophylline, class I and class III antiarrhythmics, mefloquine, diltiazem, verapamil, ergometrine, lanreotide, mexiletine, sympathomimetics, theophylline.

Drug group: β-adrenoceptor blockers (selective) (alpha-blockers)

Drug name: Atenolol

UK brand names: Tenormin

Average doses:

- 25–200 mg per day orally, 2.5 mg every 5 minutes, maximum 10 mg every 12 hours by intravenous injection or 150 mg over 20 minutes every 12 hours by intravenous infusion

(Continued)

What form does it come in: Solution for injection, oral solution, tablet

Does it interact with other medicines: Yes, the following interactions are known:

- The following drugs increase the risk of adverse events with atenolol: aminophylline, class I and class III antiarrhythmics, mefloquine, diltiazem, verapamil, ergometrine, lanreotide, mexiletine, sympathomimetics, theophylline.

Drug name: Bisoprolol fumerate

UK brand names: Cardicor

Average doses:

- 5-10 mg once daily, initial dose in heart failure 1.25 mg increasing slowly as tolerated

What form does it come in: Tablet

Does it interact with other medicines: Yes, the following interactions are known:

- As atenolol.

Drug name: Celiprolol hydrochloride

UK brand names: Celctol

Average doses:

- 200-400 mg per day

What form does it come in: Tablet

Does it interact with other medicines: Yes, the following interactions are known:

- Grapefruit juice decreases exposure.
- As atenolol.

Drug name: Esmolol hydrochloride

UK brand names: Brevibloc

Average doses:

- 50-200 micrograms/kg/minute

What form does it come in: Solution for injection

Does it interact with other medicines: Yes, the following interactions are known:

- As atenolol.

Drug name: Metoprolol tartrate

UK brand names: Betaloc

Average doses:

- Immediate release 100-300 mg per day, maximum dose 400 mg, modified release 200-400 mg per day, slow intravenous injection 5 mg, maximum dose 10-15 mg

What form does it come in: Tablet, solution for injection

Does it interact with other medicines: Yes, the following interactions are known:

- As atenolol.
- The following drugs increase exposure to metoprolol: antiandrogens, bupropion, cinacalcet, dacomitinib, duloxetine, eliglustat, HIV-protease inhibitors, mirabegron, panobinostat, SSRIs, terbinafine, vaborbactam.
- Rifamycins decrease exposure to metoprolol.

Drug name: Nebivolol

UK brand names: None

Average doses:

- 2.5-5 mg per day

(Continued)

What form does it come in: Tablet

Does it interact with other medicines: Yes, the following interactions are known:

- As atenolol.
- The following drugs increase exposure to nebivolol: antiandrogens, bupropion, cinacalcet, dacomitinib, panobinostat, SSRIs, terbinafine.

Drug group: α-adrenoceptor blockers (alpha-blockers)

Drug name: Doxazosin

UK brand names: Cardura, Doxadura, Larbex, Slocinx

Average doses:

- Immediate release 1-4 mg per day (maximum 16 mg per day), modified release 4-8 mg per day

What form does it come in: Modified release tablet, tablet

Does it interact with other medicines: Yes, the following interactions are known:

- The following drugs increase exposure to doxazosin: antifungals (azoles), cobicistat, HIV-protease inhibitors, idelalisib, clarithromycin.
- α-blockers increase risk of hypotension with phosphodiesterase type-5 inhibitors.

Drug name: Indoramin

UK brand names: Doralese Tiltab

Average doses:

- 50-200 mg per day

What form does it come in: Tablet

Does it interact with other medicines: Yes, the following interactions are known:

- The following drugs increase exposure to indoramin: mono amine oxidase inhibitors (irreversible).
- α-blockers increase risk of hypotension with phosphodiesterase type-5 inhibitors.

Drug name: Prazosin

UK brand names: Hypovase, Minipress

Average doses:

- 1-20 mg per day

What form does it come in: Tablet

Does it interact with other medicines: Yes, the following interactions are known:

- α-blockers increase risk of hypotension with phosphodiesterase type-5 inhibitors.

Drug group: α and β adrenoceptor blockers

Drug name: Carvedilol

UK brand names: None

Average doses:

- 12.5 mg initially, increasing slowly to maximum 50 mg per day

What form does it come in: Tablet

Does it interact with other medicines: Yes, the following interactions are known:

- As atenolol.
- α-blockers increase risk of hypotension with phosphodiesterase type-5 inhibitors.
- Rifamycins decrease exposure to carvedilol.

Drug name: Labetalol hydrochloride

UK brand names: Trandate

Average doses:

- Orally initially 50-100 mg up to maximum of 2.4 g per day. By intravenous injection 50 mg followed by another 50 mg after 5 minutes up to a maximum of 200 mg per course. By intravenous infusion 2 mg/minute, 50-200 mg usual dose

(Continued)

What form does it come in: Solution for injection, tablet

Does it interact with other medicines: Yes, the following interactions are known:

- As atenolol.

Drug group: Nitrates

Drug name: Glyceryl trinitrate

UK brand names: Nitrocine, Nitronal, Deponit, Minitran, Transiderm-Nitro, Glytrin, Nitrolingual, Rectogesic

Average doses:

- Sublingual tablet: One every 5 minutes up to 3 doses for treatment of angina, sublingual spray 400–800 mg prior to activity for prophylaxis of angina or 400–800 mg every 5 minutes up to 3 doses before seeking medical assistance for treatment of angina. Transdermal patch 5–15 mg per day. By intravenous infusion: 10–200 micrograms/minute up to 400 micrograms/minute

What form does it come in: Solution for infusion, sublingual tablet, transdermal patch, rectal ointment (for anal fissure, not discussed here), sublingual spray

Does it interact with other medicines: Yes, the following interactions are known:

- The following drugs increase the risk of adverse events with nitrates: local anaesthetics (prilocaine), dapsone, phosphodiesterase type-5 inhibitors.

Drug name: Isosorbide dinitrate

UK brand names: Isoket Retrad

Average doses:

- Immediate release tablets 30–160 mg per day, intravenous infusion 2–10 mg/hour up to 20 mg/hour. Modified release tablet 40–80 mg per day

What form does it come in: Modified release tablet, tablet, solution for injection, solution for infusion

Does it interact with other medicines: Yes, the following interactions are known:

- As glyceryl trinitrate.

Drug name: Isosorbide mononitrate

UK brand names: Carmil, Chemydur, Elatan LA, Imdur, Isib, Ismo Retard, Isodur Isotard, Modisai, Monomax, Monomil, Monosorb, Relosorb, Tardisc, Trangina, Xismox, Zemon

Average doses:

- Immediate release medicines 20–120 mg per day, modified release 25–120 mg per day. Half dose initially to minimise headache

What form does it come in: Modified release tablet, tablet, modified release capsule

Does it interact with other medicines: Yes, the following interactions are known:

- As glyceryl trinitrate.

Drug group: Diuretics – thiazides and related diuretics

Drug name: Bendroflumethiazide

UK brand names: Neo-Naclex

Average doses:

- 2.5 mg per day for hypertension 5–10 mg, 1–3 times a week for oedema

What form does it come in: Tablet

Does it interact with other medicines: Yes, the following interactions are known:

- The following drugs increase the risk of adverse events with thiazide diuretics: allopurinol, aspirin, calcium salts, NSAIDs, reboxetine, toremifene, vitamin D substances.
- Thiazide diuretics increase the concentration of lithium.

(Continued)

Drug name: Chlortalidone

UK brand names: None

Average doses:

- 25–50 mg per day

What form does it come in: Tablet

Does it interact with other medicines: Yes, the following interactions are known:

- As bendroflumethiazide.

Drug name: Indapamide

UK brand names: AlkapamidXL, Cardide SR, Indipam XL, Lorvacs XL, Natrilix, Rawel XL, Tensaid XL

Average doses:

- 2.5 mg per day immediate release, 1.5 mg per day modified release

Does it interact with other medicines: Yes, the following interactions are known:

- As bendroflumethiazide.

Drug name: Metolazone

UK brand names: Xaqua, Zaroxolyn

Average doses:

- 5–10 mg per day

What form does it come in: Tablet

Does it interact with other medicines: Yes, the following interactions are known:

- As bendroflumethiazide.

Drug group: Diuretics - loop

Drug name: Bumetanide

UK brand names: None

Average doses:

- 0.5-1 mg dose repeated after 6-8 hours. In severe cases of oedema 5 mg initially then increase in steps of 5 mg every 12-24 hours

What form does it come in: Oral solution, tablet

Does it interact with other medicines: Yes, the following interactions are known:

- The following drugs increase the risk of adverse events with loop diuretics: aminoglycosides, Cytomegalovirus immunoglobulins, reboxetine.
- Loop diuretics increase the concentration of lithium.

Drug name: Furosemide (Frusemide)

UK brand names: Diuresal, Frusol

Average doses:

- Orally 20-120 mg per day, by intramuscular or intravenous injection 20-50 mg then increase in steps of 20 mg every 2 hours. Doses greater than 50 mg by infusion only. Maximum 1.5 g per day

What form does it come in: Oral solution, tablet, solution for injection

Does it interact with other medicines: Yes, the following interactions are known:

- As bumetanide.
- The following drugs increase exposure to furosemide: leflunomide, dasabuvir, nitisinone, paritaprevir, teriflunomide.
- The following drugs decrease exposure to furosemide: aliskiren, antiepileptics.
- Chloral hydrate increases adverse effects with furosemide.

Drug name: Torasemide

UK brand names: Torem

Average doses:

- 2.5-5 mg per day, 40 mg per day maximum dose

(Continued)

What form does it come in: Tablet

Does it interact with other medicines: Yes, the following interactions are known:

- As bumetanide.

Drug group: Diuretics - potassium sparing

Drug name: Amiloride hydrochloride

UK brand names: None

Average doses:

- 5-10 mg per day up to 20 mg

What form does it come in: Oral solution, tablet

Does it interact with other medicines: No

Drug group: Diuretics - combined potassium sparing and loop

Drug name: Amiloride with bumetanide

UK brand names: None

Average doses:

- 1-2 tablets per day

What form does it come in: Tablet

Does it interact with other medicines: Yes, the following interactions are known:

- As bumetanide.

Drug name: Spironolactone with furosemide

UK brand names: Lasilactone

Average doses:

- 20/50-80/200 mg per day

What form does it come in: Capsule

Does it interact with other medicines: Yes, the following interactions are known:

- Spironolactone decreases the effects of antiandrogens and mitotane.
- Spironolactone increases the concentration of digoxin and lithium.
- Also see furosemide.

Drug name: Co-amilofruse

UK brand names: None

Average doses:

- 2.5/20-10/80 mg per day

What form does it come in: Tablet

Does it interact with other medicines: Yes, the following interactions are known:

- As furosemide.

Drug group: Diuretics – osmotic

Drug name: Mannitol

UK brand names: None

Average doses:

- 0.5-2 mg/kg administered over 30-60 minutes repeated 1-2 times after 4-8 hours

What form does it come in: Infusion

Does it interact with other medicines: No

DRUG CONCEPTS: ANTIARRHYTHMICS

Class I antiarrhythmic drugs (also known as membrane stabilising drugs) block the sodium channels in cardiac muscle, particularly when they are active. This means that they can help reduce over excitability and prevent premature beats, treating ventricular and supraventricular arrhythmias.

Class II antiarrhythmic drugs are the β-blockers and Class IV are CCBs (verapamil), both of which were discussed earlier. Class III antiarrhythmic drugs are amiodarone, dronedarone and sotalol. These drugs block the potassium channel in cardiac muscle cells, causing the action potential to be prolonged and therefore interrupting re-entrant tachycardias and preventing premature beats.

Some antiarrhythmic drugs are not classified into classes. Adenosine supresses conduction at the AV node and is therefore used to treat SVT caused by re-entry rhythms involving the AV node. Digoxin is a cardiac glycoside which slows the rate of the heart conduction through the AV node whilst increasing the force of contraction. Digoxin is used in the treatment of atrial fibrillation and in heart failure with reduced ejection fraction where other medication has not been successful (NICE, 2018).

GO FURTHER

Digoxin has a narrow therapeutic range and toxic levels can produce AV block and ectopic activity. The signs of digoxin poisoning are ventricular arrythmias and bradycardia that is not responsive to atropine. Digoxin should be omitted if the pulse is less than 60 beats per minute. Life-threatening toxicity can be treated with the antidote Digifab.

Drug group: Class I antiarrhythmics

Drug name: Disopyramide

UK brand names: Rythmodan

Average doses:

- Immediate release 300–800 mg per day, modified release 250–375 mg every 12 hours

What form does it come in: Modified release tablet, capsule

Does it interact with other medicines: Yes, the following interactions are known:

- The following drugs increase the risk of adverse effects with disopyramide: astemizole, cisapride, mexiletine, pentamidine, pimozide, sparfloxacin, terfenadine, thioridazone, macrolides, tricyclic antidepressants, phosphodiesterase type-5 Inhibitors, verapamil, drugs reducing potassium levels, other antiarrhythmics including beta blockers and vernakalant.
- The following drugs increase exposure to disopyramide: antifungals, cobicistat, HIV-protease inhibitors.
- The following drugs decrease exposure to disopyramide: antiandrogens, antiepileptics, rifamycin.

Drug name: Lidocaine hydrochloride

UK brand names: None

Average doses:

- 50-100 mg by intravenous injection in ventricular arrhythmias followed by further doses by intravenous infusion 1-4 mg/minute (see also UK resuscitation guidelines for emergency use)

What form does it come in: Solution for injection

Does it interact with other medicines: Yes, the following interactions are known:

- The following drugs increase the risk of adverse effects with lidocaine: astemizole, cisapride, mexiletine, pentamidine, pimozide, sparfloxacin, terfenadine, thioridazone, macrolides, tricyclic antidepressants, other antiarrhythmics, other local anaesthetics.
- The following drugs increase exposure to lidocaine: antifungals, cobicistat, HIV-protease inhibitors, ciprofloxacin, cimetidine, ranitidine, propranolol.
- The following drugs decrease exposure to disopyramide: antiandrogens, antiepileptics.
- Lidocaine increases the effects of the following drugs: suxamethonium.

(Continued)

Drug name: Flecainide acetate

UK brand names: Tambocor

Average doses:

- 100–300 mg daily

What form does it come in: Tablet

Does it interact with other medicines: Yes, the following interactions are known:

- The following drugs increase the risk of adverse effects with flecainide: clozapine, haloperidol, risperidone, mizolastine, astemizole, terfenadine mexiletine, pentamidine, pimozide, sparfloxacin, terfenadine, thioridazone, macrolides, tricyclic antidepressants, other antiarrhythmics, other local anaesthetics.
- The following drugs increase exposure to flecainide: cimetidine, antidepressants, neuroleptics, propranolol, ritonavir, antimalarials, terbinafine, SSRIs, cobicistat.
- The following drugs decrease exposure to flecainide: antiepileptics.

Drug name: Propafenone hydrochloride

UK brand names: Arythmol

Average doses:

- 150–300 mg three times a day

What form does it come in: Tablet

Does it interact with other medicines: Yes, the following interactions are known:

- The following drugs increase the risk of adverse effects with propafenone: amiodarone, local anaesthetics, clozapine, β-blockers, mexiletine, vernakalant.
- The following drugs increase exposure to propafenone: antifungals, diltiazem, verapamil, cimetidine, crizotinib, cobicistat, grapefruit juice, HIV-protease inhibitors, idelaisib, letermovir, macrolides (clarithromycin, erythromycin), nilotinib, SSRIs.
- The following drugs decrease exposure to propafenone: antiepileptics, antiandrogens, mitotane.
- Propafenone increases the effects of or exposure to: coumarins, phenindione, relugolix, tricyclic antidepressants.

Drug group: Class III antiarrhythmics

Drug name: Amiodarone hydrochloride

UK brand names: Cordarone X

Average doses:

- Orally 200 mg per day as maintenance dose, initially 200 mg three times a day, by intravenous infusion 5 mg/kg up to 1.2 mg per day (see also UK resuscitation guidelines for emergency use)

What form does it come in: Tablet, solution for injection

Does it interact with other medicines: There are a large number of interactions for this drug, some of which are included here. It should be noted that Amiodarone has a long half-life and therefore interaction can occur for weeks, even months after the last dose has been taken:

- The following drugs increase the risk of adverse effects with amiodarone: local anaesthetics, β-blockers, CCBs (diltiazem, verapamil), coumarins, chloroprocaine, ledipasvir, mexiletine, sofosbuvir, thyroid hormones, vernakalant.
- Amiodarone increases the effects or concentration of: avatrombopag, epiorenone, antiarrhythmics (propafenone, flecainide), aliskiren, antiepileptics, ciclosporin, bictegravir, colchicine, digoxin, dabigatran, erlotinuib, factor xa inhibitors, fentanyl, fidaxomicin, larotrectinib, nintedanib, pibrentasvir, relugolix, retinoids, siponimod, sirolimus, statins, sulfonylureas, talazoparib, taxanes, tacrolimus, topotecan, trametinib, velpatasvir.
- Amiodarone decreases the effects of: agalsidase alfa and beta, adenosine.
- The following drugs increase exposure to amiodarone: cobicistat, grapefruit juice, HIV-protease inhibitors, idelalisib, letermovir, lomitapide, nirmatrelvir, cimetidine, ribociclib.

Drug name: Dronedarone

UK brand names: Multaq

Average doses:

- 400 mg twice a day

(Continued)

What form does it come in: Tablet

Does it interact with other medicines: There are 625 known interactions for this drug as it is a CYP3A4, CYPA5 and CYP2D6 inhibitor, some of which are included here:

- The following drugs increase the risk of adverse effects with dronedarone: β-blockers, chloroprocaine, ergometrine, ergotamine, local anaesthetics, mexiletine, vernakalant.
- Dronedarone increases the effects or concentration of: α-blockers, epiorenone, aliskiren, antiarrhythmics (propafenone, flecainide), antihistamines (non-sedating), antipsychotics (2nd generation), benzodiazepines, bictegravir, CCBs, ciclosporin, colchicine, darifenacin, dienogest, digoxin, diltiazem, dabigatran, domperidone, dopamine receptor agonists, factor xa inhibitors, loperamide, lomitapide, methylprednisolone, monoclonal antibodies, opioids, pibrentasvir, phosphodiesterase type-5 inhibitors, pimozide, ranolazine, saxagliptin, SSRIs, statins, tacrolimus, taxanes, trazodone, topotecan, tezacaftor, tyrosine kinase inhibitors, tricyclic antidepressants, verapamil, venetoclax, vinca alkaloids, zopiclone.
- The following drugs increase exposure to dronedarone: antifungals, cimetidine, cobicistat, diltiazem, grapefruit juice, HIV-protease inhibitors, idelalisib, macrolides, neurokinin-1 antagonists, verapamil.
- The following drugs decrease exposure to dronedarone: antiandrogens, antiepileptics, NNRTIs, rifamycins, St John's Wort.

Drug group: Antiarrhythmics (other)

Drug name: Adenosine

UK brand names: Adenocor, Adenoscan

Average doses:

- 3-6 mg initially by rapid intravenous injection, followed by 6-12 mg (lower dose in patients following heart transplant)

What form does it come in: Solution for injection, solution for infusion

Does it interact with other medicines: Yes, the following interactions are known:

- Tea, coffee, chocolate, cola, xanthines decrease the effect of adenosine.
- Dipyridamole increases exposure to adenosine.

Drug name: Vernakalant

UK brand names: Brinavess

Average doses:

- 3 mg/kg reducing to 2 mg/kg, maximum 5 mg/kg per day

What form does it come in: Solution for infusion

Does it interact with other medicines: Yes, the following interactions are known:

- Not to be administered if other class I or class III antiarrhythmics have been administered in the last 4 hours.

Drug group: Cardiac glycosides

Drug name: Digoxin

UK brand names: Lanoxin

Average doses:

- Orally 62.5-250 mg per day, 0.75-1 mg by intravenous infusion as a loading dose if required

What form does it come in: Tablet, solution for infusion

Does it interact with other medicines: Yes, the following interactions are known:

- The following drugs increase the risk of adverse effects with digoxin: ceritinib, drugs that reduce potassium, pancuronium, suxamethonium, vitamin D substances.
- The following drugs increase exposure to digoxin: aminoglycosides, antifungals, amiodarone, antimalarials, berotralstat, intravenous calcium salts, carbimazole, ciclosporin, diltiazem, dronedarone, eliglustat, eplerenone, glecaprevir, HIV-protease inhibitors, indomethacin, ivacftor, ledipasvir macrolides, mirabegron, monoclonal antibodies, pibrentasvir, propafenone, ranolazine, spironolactone, ticagrelor, tolvaptan, trimethoprim, velpatasvir, verapamil, venetoclax, voxilaprevir.
- The following drugs decrease exposure to digoxin: acarbose antiandrogens antiepileptics, balsalazide, oral antacids, neomycin, penicillamine, pitolisant, rifamycins, sucralfate, St John's Wort, sulfasalazine.

DRUG CONCEPT: LIPID MODIFYING DRUGS

There are several groups of drugs which are used to treat hyperlipidaemia, the most common of which are the statins. Statins block an enzyme in the liver MHM-coA reductase which is involved in the synthesis of cholesterol. As the liver is producing less cholesterol, more low-density lipoprotein (LDL) cholesterol is taken back into the liver, reducing plasma LDL cholesterol levels. Triglyceride levels are also slightly reduced and high-density lipoprotein (HDL) cholesterol increased. Fibrates reduce triglycerides, with a smaller reduction in LDL cholesterol and rise in HDL cholesterol. Cholesterol absorption inhibitors can help reduce cholesterol absorption from the duodenum. This can be used in conjunction with a statin or alone when a statin is contraindicated, along with dietary modification. Proprotein convertase subtilisin/kexin type-9 (PCSK9) inhibitors act on the enzyme which deactivates LDL receptors in the liver. LDL receptors allow the reuptake and recycling of LDL cholesterol in the liver, reducing plasma levels, therefore inhibiting this enzyme encourages this process.

Drug group: Lipid modifying drugs (cholesterol absorption inhibitors)

Drug name: Ezetimibe

UK brand names: Ezetrol

Average doses:

- 10 mg per day

What form does it come in: Tablet

Does it interact with other medicines: Yes, the following interactions are known:

- Ciclosporin increases exposure to ezetimbe.
- Fibrates increase risk of gall stones.

Drug group: Lipid modifying drugs (fibrates)

Drug name: Bezafibrate

UK brand names: Bezalip, Fibrazate XL

Average doses:

- Immediate release 200 mg three times a day, modified release 400 mg daily

What form does it come in: Modified release tablet, tablet

Does it interact with other medicines: Yes, the following interactions are known:

- The following drugs increase the risk of adverse effects with bezafibrate: acipimox, ciclosporin, colchicine, daptomycin, ezetimibe, insulin, statins, sulfonylureas.
- Fibrates increase the anticoagulant effects of: coumarins, phenindione.
- Fibrates reduce the efficacy of: ursodeoxycholic acid.

Drug name: Ciprofibrate

UK brand names: None

Average doses:

- 100 mg per day

What form does it come in: Tablet

Does it interact with other medicines: Yes, the following interactions are known:

- As bezafibrate (not ciclosporin).

Drug name: Fenofibrate

UK brand names: Supralip, Lipantil

Average doses:

- 160-267 mg per day

What form does it come in: Capsule, tablet

Does it interact with other medicines: Yes, the following interactions are known:

- As bezafibrate.

(Continued)

Drug name: Gemfibrozil

UK brand names: Lopid

Average doses:

- 0.9–1.2 g per day

What form does it come in: Tablet

Does it interact with other medicines: Yes, the following interactions are known:

- As bezafibrate (not ciclosporin).
- Gemfibrozil increases the concentration/exposure to: antiandrogens, dabrafenib, dasabuvir, irinotecan, letermovir, repaglinide, montelukast, ozanimod, pioglitazone, retinoids, selexipag, paclitaxel.

Drug group: Lipid modifying drugs (statins)

Drug name: Atorvastatin

UK brand names: Lipitor

Average doses:

- 10–80 mg per day

What form does it come in: Tablet, chewable tablet

Does it interact with other medicines: Yes, the following interactions are known:

- The following drugs increase the risk of adverse effects with atorvastatin: acipimox, colchicine, daptomycin, fibrates, fusidate, nicotinic acid.
- The following drugs increase exposure to atorvastatin: antifungals amiodarone, ceftobiprole, ciclosporin, cilostazol, cobicistat, crizotinib, diltiazem, dronedarone, elbasvir, eltrombopag, fostemsavir, glecaprevir, grapefruit juice, grazoprevir, HIV-protease inhibitors, idelalisib, imatinib, ledipasvir, leflunomide, letermovir, lomitapide, macrolides, neurokinin-1 receptor antagonists, nilotinib, osmertinib, pibrentasvir, ranolazine, regorafenib, tedizolid, teriflunomide, tepotinib, venetoclax, verapamil, voxilaprevir.
- The following drugs decrease exposure to atorvastatin: antiandrogens, antiepileptics, bosentan, monoclonal antibodies, NNRTIs, rifamycins, St John's Wort.
- Atorvastatin increases exposure to: aliskiren.

Drug name: Fluvastatin

UK brand names: Dorisin XL, Lescol XL, Nandovar XL

Average doses:

- 20-80 mg per day

What form does it come in: Modified release tablet, capsule

Does it interact with other medicines: Yes, the following interactions are known:

- The following drugs increase the risk of adverse effects with atorvastatin: acipimox, colchicine, daptomycin, fibrates, fusidate, nicotinic acid.
- The following drugs increase exposure to atorvastatin: antifungals, amiodarone, ceftobiprole, ciclosporin, elbasvir, eltrombopag, fostemsavir, glecaprevir, grapefruit juice, grazoprevir, ledipasvir, leflunomide, letermovir, mifepristone, pibrentasvir, regorafenib, tedizolid, teriflunomide, venetoclax, verapamil, voxilaprevir.
- The following drugs decrease exposure to atorvastatin: antiandrogens, bosentan, rifamycins.

Drug name: Pravastatin sodium

UK brand names: None

Average doses:

- 10-40 mg per day

What form does it come in: Tablet

Does it interact with other medicines: Yes, the following interactions are known:

- The following drugs increase the risk of adverse effects with pravastatin: acipimox, colchicine, daptomycin, fibrates, fusidate, nicotinic acid.
- The following drugs increase exposure to pravastatin: antifungals, bempedoic acid, ceftobiprole, ciclosporin, crizitinib, elexacaftor, eltrombopag, glecaprevir, ledipasvir, leflunomide, letermovir, Macrolides, pibrentasvir, ribociclib, teriflunomide, venetoclax, voxilaprevir.
- The following drugs decrease exposure to pravastatin: antiandrogens.
- Pravastatin increases the effects of: coumarins.

(Continued)

Drug name: Rosuvastatin

UK brand names: Crestor

Average doses:

- 5-40 mg per day

What form does it come in: Tablet

Does it interact with other medicines: Yes, the following interactions are known:

- The following drugs increase the risk of adverse effects with rosuvastatin: acipimox, colchicine, daptomycin, fibrates, fusidate, nicotinic acid.
- The following drugs increase exposure to rosuvastatin: antifungals, ceftobiprole, ciclosporin, elbasvir, eltrombopag, fostamatinib, glecaprevir, grazoprevir, HIV-protease inhibitors, ledipasvir, leflunomide, letermovir, mifepristone, osimertinib, pibrentasvir, regorafenib, ribociclib, tedizolid, tivozanib, teriflunomide, venetoclax, voxilaprevir.
- The following drugs decrease exposure to rosuvastatin: antiandrogens, oral antacids.
- Pravastatin increases the effects of: coumarins.

Drug name: Simvastatin

UK brand names: Simvador, Zocor

Average doses:

- 20-80 mg per day

What form does it come in: Oral suspension, tablet

Does it interact with other medicines: Yes, the following interactions are known:

- The following drugs increase the risk of adverse effects with simvastatin: acipimox, colchicine, daptomycin, fibrates, fusidate, nicotinic acid.
- The following drugs increase exposure to simvastatin: antifungals, amiodarone, bempedoic acid, ceftobiprole, ciclosporin, cobicistat, crizotinib, dasabuvir, diltiazem, dronedarone, elbasvir, eltrombopag, fostamatinib, fostemsavir, glecaprevir, grapefruit juice, grazoprevir, ledipasvir, leflunomide, letermovir, lomitapide, mifepristone, pibrentasvir, ranolazine, regorafenib, ribociclib, roxadustat, tedizolid, teriflunomide, ticagrelor, velpatasvir, venetoclax, verapamil, voxilaprevir.
- The following drugs decrease exposure to simvastatin: antiandrogens, antiepileptics, bosentan, rifamycins, St John's Wort.

Drug group: Lipid modifying drugs (PCSK9 inhibitors)

Drug name: Alirocumab

UK brand names: Praluent

Average doses:

- 75-150 mg every two weeks or 300 mg every four weeks

What form does it come in: Solution for injection

Does it interact with other medicines: No

Drug name: Evolocumab

UK brand names: Repatha Sureclick

Average doses:

- 140-420 mg every two weeks

What form does it come in: Solution for injection

Does it interact with other medicines: No

DRUG CONCEPT: BLOOD CLOTTING

The next section will discuss drugs that affect blood clotting. Vitamin K is required for the production of clotting factors II, VII, IX and X. Warfarin (a coumarin derivative) is a vitamin K antagonist and therefore reduces the production of these clotting factors. The response of patients to warfarin varies widely and therefore the dose is altered in line with the international normalised ratio (INR) blood results. Oral thrombin inhibitors and factor Xa inhibitors are increasingly used as they do not require titration or monitoring through blood tests. Heparin and low-molecular weight heparins or heparinoids are given by injection or intravenously. They work by potentiating antithrombin III which inactivates factor Xa and thrombin, although heparinoids have less effect on thrombin than heparin. Heparin dose needs to be monitored through a blood test, activated partial thromboplastin time.

Platelets are also required for blood clotting and several drugs affect platelet activation and aggregation. Aspirin, ADP antagonists such as clopidogrel and prasugrel, glycoprotein IIb/IIIa inhibitors and epoprostenol all inhibit platelet activation and aggregation but in slightly different parts of the process.

Once a clot is formed, a fibrinolytic drug is required to break it down. These drugs increase the conversion of plasminogen to plasmin which digests fibrin and breaks down clots. Steptokinase is a plasminogen activating protein which is derived from bacteria, but causes antibodies to be formed by the recipient and can therefore only be given once. Tissue-type plasminogen activators (tPA) are more active on fibrin bound plasminogen and are therefore more clot selective. They do not generally cause antibody formation. These drugs are used to treat myocardial infarction and ischaemic stroke. Transexamic acid inhibits plasminogen activation and can be given to reduce bleeding and counteract streptokinase and tPA.

Drug group: Antiplatelet drugs

Drug name: Aspirin (acetylsalicylic acid)

UK brand names: Nu-Seals, Danamep, Disprin

Average doses:

- 75–150 mg per day for secondary prevention; 300 mg for ischaemic stroke and myocardial infarction; 300–900 mg 4–6 hourly up to 4 g per day for pain; 75–150 mg for prevention of preeclampsia for women at risk

What form does it come in: Gastro-resistant tablet, tablet, suppository, dispersible tablet

Does it interact with other medicines: Yes, the following interactions are known (with high doses):

- Increased risk of bleeding if administered with other drugs with anticoagulant or antiplatelet effects.
- Increased adverse effects when given with the following: acetazolamide, bismuth, bisphosphonates, corticosteroids, daptomycin, erlotinib, deferasirox, methotrexate, nicorandil, NRTIs, selumetinib, thiazide diuretics.
- Aspirin increases exposure to: edoxaban, pemetrexed.
- Oral antacids decrease absorption of aspirin.

Drug name: Cilostazol

UK brand names: Pletal

Average doses:

- 100 mg twice daily

What form does it come in: Tablet

Does it interact with other medicines: Yes, the following interactions are known:

- Increased risk of bleeding if administered with other drugs with anticoagulant or antiplatelet effects, selumetinib.
- The following increase exposure to cilostazol: antifungals, cobicistat, HIV-protease inhibitors, idelalisib, macrolides, moclobemide, proton pump inhibitors, SSRIs.
- Cilostazol increases exposure to: cladribine, lomitapide, statins.
- The following may alter the effects of cilotazole: anti-androgens, antiepileptics, mitotane, rifamycins, St John's Wort.

Drug name: Clopidogrel

UK brand names: Plavix

Average doses:

- Initially 300 mg then 75 mg per day for up to 12 months

What form does it come in: Tablet

Does it interact with other medicines: Yes, the following interactions are known:

- Increased risk of bleeding if administered with other drugs with anticoagulant or antiplatelet effects.
- Clopidogrel increases exposure to: antiandrogens, dabrafenib, montelukast, ozanimod, pioglitazone, selexipag, repaglinide, retinoids.
- The following decrease the effects of clopidogrel: antifungals, cobicistat, grapefruit juice, moclobemide, proton pump inhibitors, ritonavir, SSRIs, statins, paclitaxel.
- Rifampicin increases the effects of clopidogrel.

Drug name: Dipyridamole

UK brand names: Attia, Ofcram PR

Average doses:

- Modified release 400 mg per day, immediate release 300–600 mg per day

(Continued)

What form does it come in: Oral suspension, modified release capsule, tablet

Does it interact with other medicines: Yes, the following interactions are known:

- Increased risk of bleeding if administered with other drugs with anticoagulant or antiplatelet effects.
- Dipyridamole increases exposure to adenosine.
- The following drugs decrease absorption of dipyridamole: h2 receptor antagonists, proton pump inhibitors, oral antacids.

Drug group: Factor xa inhibitors

Drug name: Apixaban

UK brand names: Eliquis

Average doses:

- 2.5–5 mg per day for prophylaxis, 10 mg reducing to 5 mg per day for treatment of deep vein thrombosis (DVT) or pulmonary embolus (PE)

What form does it come in: Tablet

Does it interact with other medicines: Yes, the following interactions are known:

- Increased risk of bleeding if administered with other drugs with anticoagulant or antiplatelet effects.
- The following drugs increase exposure to apixaban: amiodarone, dronedarone, antifungals (azoles), ciclosporin, cobicistat, HIV-protease inhibitors, idelalisib, lapatinib, macrolides, ranolazine rifamycins, vandetanib, vemurafenib, verapamil.
- The following drugs decrease exposure to apixaban: antiandrogens, antiepileptics, mitotane, St John's Wort.

Drug name: Edoxaban

UK brand names: Lixiana

Average doses:

- 30–60 mg per day

What form does it come in: Tablet

Does it interact with other medicines: Yes, the following interactions are known:

- Increased risk of bleeding if administered with other drugs with anticoagulant or antiplatelet effects.
- The following drugs increase exposure to edoxaban: abrocitinib, amiodarone, berotralstat, dronedarone, antifungals (azoles), certinib, ciclosporin, cobicistat, eliglustat, HIV-protease inhibitors, ibrutinib, ivacaftor, lapatinib, lorlatinib, macrolides, mirabegron, neratinib, olaparib, osimertinib, pemigatinib, pibrentasvir, pitolisant, ranolazine rifamycins, sotorasib, tepotinib, tucatinib, vandetanib, vemurafenib, velpatasvir, venetoclax, verapamil, voxilaprevir.
- The following drugs decrease exposure to edoxaban: antiepileptics, St John's Wort.

Drug name: Fondaparinux sodium

UK brand names: Arixtra

Average doses:

- 2.5 mg per day by subcutaneous injection. For treatment of DVT or PE 5-10 mg per day by subcutaneous injection

What form does it come in: Solution for injection

Does it interact with other medicines: No

Drug name: Rivaroxaban

UK brand names: Xarelto

Average doses:

- 2.5-20 mg per day

What form does it come in: Tablet

Does it interact with other medicines: Yes, the following interactions are known:

- As edoxaban.

Drug group: Heparins and heparinoids

Drug name: Danaparoid sodium

UK brand names: None

Average doses:

- 750 units twice a day for 7-10 days prior to surgery for prophylaxis. For treatment of thromboembolic disease in patients with history of heparin induced thrombocytopenia 1250-3750 units initially then 400-200 units per hour by continuous infusion for five days

What form does it come in: Solution for injection

Does it interact with other medicines: Yes, the following interactions are known:

- Increased risk of bleeding if administered with other drugs with anticoagulant or antiplatelet effects.

Drug name: Dalteparin sodium

UK brand names: Fragmin

Average doses:

- Treatment of DVT or PE 200-400 units/kg per day. For prophylaxis in medical and surgical patients 2500 to 5000 units per day

What form does it come in: Solution for injection

Does it interact with other medicines: Yes, the following interactions are known:

- Increased risk of bleeding if administered with other drugs with anticoagulant or antiplatelet effects.

Drug name: Enoxaparin sodium

UK brand names: Arovi, Clexane, Inhixa

Average doses:

- 20-40 mg per day for prophylaxis; 40-100 mg twice daily for treatment of DVT or PE, or 1-1.5 mg/kg every 12-24 hours

What form does it come in: Solution for injection

Does it interact with other medicines: Yes, the following interactions are known:

- Increased risk of bleeding if administered with other drugs with anticoagulant or antiplatelet effects.

Drug name: Heparin

UK brand names: None

Average doses:

- Treatment of DVT or PE 5000-10,000 units initially followed by 18 units/kg/hour by continuous infusion. For prophylaxis in medical and surgical patients 5000 units every 8-12 hours

What form does it come in: Solution for injection, intravenous flush, infusion

Does it interact with other medicines: Yes, the following interactions are known:

- Increased risk of bleeding if administered with other drugs with anticoagulant or antiplatelet effects.
- Ranibizumab.

Drug name: Tinzaparin sodium

UK brand names: Innohep

Average doses:

- 3500-4500 units per day for prophylaxis, 175 units/kg daily for treatment of DVT or PE

What form does it come in: Solution for injection

Does it interact with other medicines: Yes, the following interactions are known:

- Increased risk of bleeding if administered with other drugs with anticoagulant or antiplatelet effects.

Drug group: Thrombin inhibitors

Drug name: Argatroban monohydrate

UK brand names: Exembol

Average doses:

- 2 micrograms/kg/minute up to 10 micrograms/kg/minute

What form does it come in: Solution for infusion

Does it interact with other medicines: Yes, the following interactions are known:

- Ranibizumab increases risk of bleeding
- Increased risk of bleeding if administered with other drugs with anticoagulant or antiplatelet effects.

Drug name: Bivalirudin

UK brand names: None

Average doses:

- Initially 100 micrograms/kg then 250 micrograms/kg/hour for up to 72 hours. Doses vary in patients undergoing percutaneous coronary intervention

What form does it come in: Powder for solution for infusion

Does it interact with other medicines: Yes, the following interactions are known:

- Ranibizumab increases risk of bleeding
- Increased risk of bleeding if administered with other drugs with anticoagulant or antiplatelet effects.

Drug name: Dabigatran etexilate

UK brand names: Pradaxa

Average doses:

- For prophylaxis 75–110 mg initially prior to surgery then 150-220 mg once to twice daily. For treatment of DVT or PE 110-150 mg twice a day

What form does it come in: Capsule

Does it interact with other medicines: Yes, the following interactions are known:

- Increased risk of bleeding if administered with other drugs with anticoagulant or antiplatelet effects.

Drug group: Vitamin K antagonists

Drug name: Acenocoumarol

UK brand names: Sinthrome

Average doses:

- 2-4 mg daily initially then 1-8 mg daily adjusted to INR

What form does it come in: Tablet

Does it interact with other medicines: There are a large number of interactions with this drug, some of which are included here:

- Increased risk of bleeding if administered with other drugs with anticoagulant or antiplatelet effects: cephalosporins, tyrosine kinase inhibitors, ranibizumab.
- The following will decrease the effects of acenocoumarol: bosentan, dietary vitamin K and enteral feeds containing vitamin K, dabrafenib, glucosamine, griseofulvin, HIV-protease inhibitors, mercaptopurine, neurokinin-1 receptor antagonists, rifamycins, St Johns Wort, sucralfate, teriflunomide.
- The following increases the effects of or exposure of acenocoumarol: pomegranate juice, alcohol, amiodarone, antifungals, antibiotics, capecitabine, cimetidine, ceritinib, corticosteroids, disulfiram, erlotinib, fibrates, fluorouracil, gefitinib, glucagon, ivermectin, leflunomide, nandrolone, nitisinone, NNRIs, oxymetholone, oral antidiabetics, paracetamol, propafenone, statins, sulfonamindes, tamoxifen, tegafur, toremifene.
- The following decrease exposure to acenocoumarol: antiandrogens, antiepileptics, azathioprine, elvitegravir, pitolisant.

(Continued)

Drug name: Phenindione

UK brand names: None

Average doses:

- 200 mg on day one, 100 mg on day two then 50–150 mg daily adjusted to INR

What form does it come in: Tablet
Does it interact with other medicines: Yes, the following interactions are known:

- Increased risk of bleeding if administered with other drugs with anticoagulant or antiplatelet effects: cephalosporins, tyrosine kinase inhibitors, ranibizumab.
- The following will decrease the effects of phenindione: dietary vitamin K and enteral feeds containing vitamin K, dabrafenib.
- The following increases the effects of or exposure to phenindione: antifungals, cimetidine, ceritinib, corticosteroids, disulfiram, erlotinib, fibrates, nandrolone, oxymetholone, paracetamol, penicillins, propafenone, statins, tetracyclines, tigecycline.

Drug name: Warfarin

UK brand names: None

Average doses:

- Initially 5–10 mg then 3–9 mg daily adjusted to INR

What form does it come in: Tablet, oral suspension

Does it interact with other medicines: Yes, the following interactions are known:

- As acenocoumarol.
- The following increases the effects of or exposure to warfarin: cobicistat, cranberry juice, ivacaftor, lomitapide, mifepristone, venetoclax.
- Metreleptin, mexiletine.
- The following decrease exposure to of effects of warfarin: letermovir, obeticholic acid, rifaximin.

Drug group: Antithrombotic drugs – glycoprotein IIb/IIIa inhibitors

Drug name: Eptifibatide

UK brand names: Integrilin

Average doses:

- Initially 180 micrograms/kg then 2 micrograms/kg/minute for up to 72 to 96 hours

What form does it come in: Solution for injection, solution for infusion

Does it interact with other medicines: Yes, the following interactions are known:

- Increased risk of bleeding if administered with other drugs with anticoagulant or antiplatelet effects.

Drug name: Tirofiban

UK brand names: Aggrastat

Average doses:

- Initially 400 nanograms/kg/minute for 30 minutes then 100 nanograms/kg/minute for at least 48 hours

What form does it come in: Solution for infusion, infusion

Does it interact with other medicines: Yes, the following interactions are known:

- Increased risk of bleeding if administered with other drugs with anticoagulant or antiplatelet effects.

Drug group: Antithrombotic drugs – fibrinolytic

Drug name: Alteplase

UK brand names: Actilyse

(Continued)

Average doses:

- 10-15 mg initially by injection, followed by an infusion, dose dependent on weight, regimen and condition

What form does it come in: Powder and solvent for injection, powder and solvent for infusion

Does it interact with other medicines: Yes, the following interactions are known:

- Increased risk of bleeding if administered with other drugs with anticoagulant or antiplatelet effects.

Drug name: Streptokinase

UK brand names: None

Average doses:

- For myocardial infarction 1,500,000 units over 60 minutes. For DVT, arterial thrombosis or PE 250,000 units to be given over 30 minutes then 100,000 units every hours for 12 hours to five days depending on condition being treated

What form does it come in: Powder for solution for infusion

Does it interact with other medicines: Yes, the following interactions are known:

- Increased risk of bleeding if administered with other drugs with anticoagulant or antiplatelet effects.

Drug name: Tenecteplase

UK brand names: Metalyse

Average doses:

- 30-50 mg given over ten seconds

What form does it come in: Powder and solvent for infusion

Does it interact with other medicines: Yes, the following interactions are known:

- Increased risk of bleeding if administered with other drugs with anticoagulant or antiplatelet effects.

DRUGS FOR THE CARDIOVASCULAR SYSTEM IN PREGNANCY AND BREASTFEEDING

There are many changes to the body during pregnancy, particularly within the circulatory system. This puts a deal of strain on the pregnant person and any underlying pathology or vulnerability may be uncovered or in pregnancy may be the cause of the circulatory problem such as in preeclampsia. It is important, both for the mother and foetus, that circulation is maintained and that any symptoms are treated. However, as always there is a balance of risk and minimum amounts of medication should be used to treat any condition and cardiology advice sought. Some drugs highlighted in this chapter are not suitable for use in pregnancy due to the harm that they can cause (Joint Formulary Committee, 2024). Where possible arrythmias should be treated by electrical cardioversion or vagal manoeuvres. Digoxin can be used in pregnancy along with beta blockers and verapamil, although betablockers have been associated with intrauterine growth retardation (Helpern et al., 2019).

ACE inhibitors are contraindicated, especially in the second and third trimesters as they can cause foetal death, however the condition of the pregnant person must be considered and use reserved for hypertension that cannot be controlled by any other means. The risk of foetal death is even higher with angiotensin II inhibitors. Diuretics potentially reduce blood flow to the placenta and aldosterone inhibitors can potentially affect the development of male foetuses, but their use may be required and preferable to ACE inhibitors and angiotensin II inhibitors in hypertension and heart failure (UKTIS, 2023). Labetalol is licensed for use in the UK for hypertension in pregnancy.

Vitamin K antagonists cross the placenta and cause foetal abnormalities and placental, foetal or neonatal haemorrhage. Low molecular weight heparins do not cross the placenta (Helpern et al., 2019). Low dose aspirin is prescribed in pregnancy and is considered safe, although higher doses can cause premature closure of the ductus arteriosus (Helpern et al., 2019). Fibrates are potentially teratogenic and it is advised that statins are stopped three months before pregnancy is planned (UKTIS, 2023).

On delivery of the baby, in some cases the strain on the circulatory system may be reduced and treatment either reduced or not required. However ongoing and pre-existing conditions will need to be treated appropriately. Amiodarone should be avoided if breastfeeding as it is present in significant amounts in breast milk (Chizuko and Yoshimatsu, 2019).

LEARNING FROM A CASE STUDY: TEST YOUR KNOWLEDGE

Mohammad is a 65-year-old man whose family originated from Pakistan. He has a history of type 2 diabetes, hypertension and had a myocardial infarction two years ago which has resulted in a stage 3 heart failure with a reduced ejection fraction and angina. Mohammad does not drink alcohol or smoke but has a BMI of 32 and central obesity. He also has raised LDL cholesterol and triglycerides. He finds exercising difficult because of his heart failure and is now retired from his job as an office manager and has become rather socially isolated.

He has been prescribed lisinopril but is finding that he has a cough which he cannot tolerate. He is also prescribed metformin, simvastatin, low dose aspirin, carvedilol, bumetanide and a glyceryl trinitrate spray.

1   What risk factors does Mohammad have for cardiovascular disease?
2   What alternative treatment could Mohammad have to replace the lisinopril?
3   Reviewing Mohammad's medications, what types of drugs are they and what do they do to help his conditions?
4   What other support would you suggest for Mohammad to improve his quality of life?

IF I REMEMBER 5 THINGS FROM THIS CHAPTER:

1   Cardiovascular disease has a major impact in terms of morbidity and mortality as well as costs to the health service and to those who are affected.
2   Many of the conditions co-occur, cause or exacerbate each other and therefore drug treatments can be complex.
3   Many of the drugs have many interactions and care must be taken.
4   Pregnancy may exacerbate cardiovascular disorders and drug treatment should balance the risk to the pregnant person and the foetus.
5   Lifestyle factors must also be considered alongside any surgical, electrical or drug treatment.

ANSWERS TO CASE STUDY QUESTIONS

1   Mohammad is of South Asian origin and therefore at higher risk for cardiovascular disease and at an earlier age. He is also overweight, has high cholesterol, type 2 diabetes and is hypertensive. These factors increase the likelihood of atherosclerosis, myocardial infarction, stroke, peripheral vascular disease and heart failure.
2   As Mohammad is not tolerating an ACE inhibitor, he should be offered an angiotensin II inhibitor.
3   Metformin – a biguanide which reduces the reduction of insulin resistance (see Chapter 4). Simvastatin – a statin to reduce blood cholesterol (must not drink grapefruit juice). Aspirin – antiplatelet to reduce the likelihood of blood clots associated with atherosclerosis. Carvedilol – a β-blocker licensed for use in heart failure to help. Bumetanide – a loop diuretic to reduce pulmonary and systemic oedema caused by heart failure. Glyceryl trinitrate – a nitrate which causes vasodilation of coronary arteries to relieve angina.
4   Mohammad would benefit from support from a multidisciplinary heart failure team including exercise and rehabilitation. He may also benefit from a support group to meet with others who have the same chronic condition. Depression is also common with chronic conditions such as heart failure, especially when it has life-changing and life-limiting implications. He may benefit from discussing this with his GP or heart failure specialist.

REFERENCES AND RECOMMENDED READING

Ashelford, S., Raynsford, J. and Taylor, V. (2019) *Pathophysiology and Pharmacology in Nursing* (2nd edn). London: Sage Publications.

Chizuko, A.K. and Yoshimatsu, J. (2019) Pharmacological treatment for cardiovascular disease during pregnancy and lactation. *Journal of Cardiology, 73*(5): 363–369.

Datapharm (2023) *Electronic Medicines Compendium*. Available at: www.medicines.org.uk/emc

Gov.uk (2017) Health matters: Combating high blood pressure. Available at: www.gov.uk/government/publications/health-matters-combating-high-blood-pressure/health-matters-combating-high-blood-pressure

Haque, M. (2020) Government must prioritise heart health in the Budget. Avialable at: https://www.bhf.org.uk/what-we-do/news-from-the-bhf/news-archive/2020/march/government-prioritise-heart-health-budget

Helpern, D., Weinberg, C., Pinnelas, R., Mehta-Lee, S., Economy, E. and Valente, A. (2019) Use of medication for cardiovascular disease during pregnancy. *Journal of the American College of Cardiology, 73*(4): 457–476. https://doi.org/10.1016/j.jacc.2018.10.075

Joint Formulary Committee (2024) British National Formulary. Available at: https://bnf.nice.org.uk/

Miller, A.J. and Arnold, A.C. (2022) The renin-angiotensin system and cardiovascular autonomic control in aging. *Peptides, 150*: 170733.

National Institute for Health and Care Excellence (NICE) (2022) Hypertension in adults: Diagnosis and management. Available at: www.nice.org.uk/guidance/ng136/chapter/Recommendations#starting-antihypertensive-drug-treatment

National Institute for Health and Care Excellence (NICE) (2018) Chronic heart failure in adults: Diagnosis and management Available at: www.nice.org.uk/guidance/ng106/chapter/Recommendations#monitoring-treatment-for-all-types-of-heart-failure

Office for Nationals Statistics (2022) Avoidable mortality in Great Britain: 2020 Available at: https://www.ons.gov.uk/peoplepopulationandcommunity/healthandsocialcare/causesofdeath/bulletins/avoidablemortalityinenglandandwales/2020

Palmer, S. J. (2020) The rising cost of medication in the UK. *British Journal of Cardiac Nursing 15*(1): 1-4.

Ritter, J.M., Flower, R., Henderson, H., Kong Loke, Y., MacEwan, D. and Rang, H.P. (2020) *Rang and Dale's Pharmacology* (9th edn). Edinburgh: Elsevier.

UK Teratology Information Service (2023) UKTIS monographs. Available at: https://uktis.org/mongraphs

7 MEDICINES FOR PAIN

SHEILA CUNNINGHAM

AFTER READING THIS CHAPTER YOU WILL BE ABLE TO:

- Describe the concept of pain, pain pathways and principles of pain management.
- Outline what is meant by the 'analgesic ladder' giving examples of medicines within this.
- Consider the risks and benefits of analgesia.
- Apply knowledge around analgesia for pain management to support clinical decision making.

OVERVIEW

Pain is a sensation many of us have experienced at some point. It is challenging to describe and even to measure, however for anyone who experiences pain they know what it is. It ought to be remembered that pain is not a condition but a symptom, and as such the cause should be investigated. Pain is often described as having many or several dimensions; it is complex and requires holistic and ongoing assessment and effective management (International Association for the Study of Pain (IASP), 2022). In a revised definition of pain, Raja et al, 2020 state it is: 'an unpleasant sensory and emotional experience associated with, or resembling that associated with, actual or potential tissue damage' (Raja et al, 2020: 1976) or, more simply, pain is what the patient describes and feels. Previously the pain sensation was termed 'nociception' referring to the noxious or unpleasant nature of it, however IASP (2022: 1) assert that pain is more complex and cannot be inferred 'solely from activity in sensory neurons'. These definitions make it clear that tissue damage is not necessarily required to experience pain. It can be medically induced (i.e. surgery) and also influenced by physical, social, psychological and emotional factors – termed multidimensional. It is also conceptualised or experienced by people through life experiences. Pain is feared and may contribute to slowing healing processes due to stress responses invoked. However, pain is individual to the person experiencing it. Furthermore, individuals may respond differently to different medicines, hence the need for attention in prescribing and administering these medicines or drugs, and monitoring effects, interactions and any adjustments which may be needed. Pain is a symptom and when the underlying cause is established (if possible) and treated then pain may be managed without analgesics, e.g. reducing inflammation, relieving pressure etc.

There have been many developments to enable pain relief or control. Pain medications work in a variety of ways so a grasp of the underpinning mechanisms of pain is important. Physiologically nociception or a noxious (unpleasant) sensation can be described as acute (sudden severe onset) or chronic (longer term, persisting and penetrating) or in terms of location (i.e. headache) or cause (i.e. inflammatory from tissue damage). Pain is transmitted via the nervous system and interpreted within the brain. Acute pain is usually more rapid in onset, more intense and often easier to control with analgesia until the cause is found and addressed. Chronic pain is more insidious (unsure of onset) but builds in intensity and is relentless – 'quality of life' threatening rather than life threatening – often leading to suffering or distress, and is a challenge to effectively manage. There are further classification types referred to as nociceptive, non-nociceptive or inflammatory (see Figure 7.1).

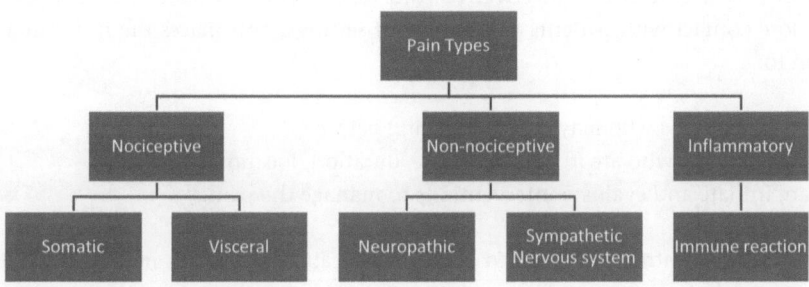

Figure 7.1 Classifications of pain

- **Nociceptive pain:** represents the normal response to noxious insult or injury of tissues such as skin, muscles, visceral organs, joints, tendons or bones (e.g. musculoskeletal). This may be acute or chronic.
- **Non-nociceptive or neuropathic pain:** caused by a primary lesion or disease in the sensory nervous system (e.g. nerve degeneration, nerve infection).
- **Inflammatory pain:** a result of activation and sensitisation of the nociceptive pain pathway by a variety of chemicals released at a site of tissue inflammation (e.g. burns, arthritis).

The IASP (2022) identify several terms associated with pain which may be used in the communication between health professionals which are worth knowing. A few are given in Table 7.1.

There are well-recognised pain disorders that are not easily classifiable. Whilst understanding of their mechanisms might be unclear there might be specific therapies established for those disorders. They include cancer pain, migraine and other primary headaches, and widespread pain of the fibromyalgia type. Treatment for the primary condition causing the pain may also enable reduction or management of the pain in addition to specific analgesic drug therapy.

Table 7.1   Terms associated with pain

Term	Explanation
Allodynia	Pain due to a stimulus that does not normally provoke pain, for example heightened sensitivity following a burn.
Hyperalgesia	Increased pain from a stimulus that normally provokes pain.
Neuralgia	Pain in the distribution of a nerve or nerves.
Neuritis	Inflammation of a nerve or nerves.
Nociception	The neural process of receiving and interpreting a sensation as a noxious stimulus.
Pain threshold	The minimum intensity of a stimulus that is perceived as painful.
Pain tolerance level	The maximum intensity of a pain-producing stimulus that a person is willing to accept in a given situation.

Nurses play a critical role in effective pain assessment and management because they are in close contact with patients in a variety of settings. This places the nurse in a unique position to:

- Identify patients who may be experiencing pain
- Assess patients who are in pain for cause, duration, location and effect
- Plan, initiate and evaluate interventions to manage the pain.

As nurses are so central they need to be knowledgeable about pain mechanisms; different types or sources of pain; potential barriers to effective pain relief and control; and a range of available methods for relieving pain. Verbal report and description is only one way to express pain and pain should not be assumed to not be present if the person is unable to express it verbally (IASP, 2022). The goals of pain management are to a large extent determined by those experiencing pain themselves.

DRUG TREATMENTS

There are a broad range of pain medications collectively termed 'analgesia' but also other medications which can used alongside to 'boost' or support the effectiveness of the analgesia called 'adjuvants'. An example of this can be seen in preparations such as 'paracetamol extra' which contains paracetamol (analgesia) and caffeine (stimulant) to enhance pain relief. The 'ideal analgesia' will relieve pain, work rapidly, act over an extended period of time, minimise interruption/return by pain (breakthrough pain), be well tolerated with minimal side effects and produce analgesia over a wide range of pain types. At present there are no 'ideal analgesics' since those available fulfil only some of these features. Patients are individuals and so their responses to analgesia may be variable, including their level of pain relief and any emergent side effects.

A wide range of drugs are used to manage pain – these can be broadly divided into 'opioid' and 'non-opioid' analgesics. Whilst originally devised for analgesic management of cancer pain, the World Health Organisation's (WHO) in 1986 introduced an 'analgesic ladder' which proposed using an escalation of analgesic drug types to manage pain which ought be prompt, regular, oral (if possible) and increasing in potency. If the patient does not experience pain relief on one 'step' of the ladder they move to the next. This ladder has three steps: step 1: non-opioids; step 2: weak opioids; and step 3: strong opioids (see Figure 7.2). This approach is also advocated by NICE (2021) in their clinical knowledge summaries.

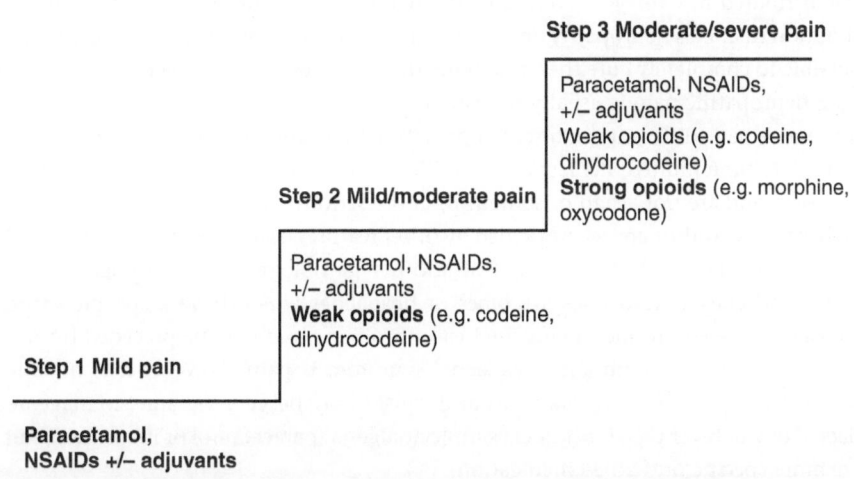

Step 3 Moderate/severe pain

Paracetamol, NSAIDs,
+/– adjuvants
Weak opioids (e.g. codeine,
dihydrocodeine)
Strong opioids (e.g. morphine,
oxycodone)

Step 2 Mild/moderate pain

Paracetamol, NSAIDs,
+/– adjuvants
Weak opioids (e.g. codeine,
dihydrocodeine)

Step 1 Mild pain

**Paracetamol,
NSAIDs +/– adjuvants**

Figure 7.2 WHO (1986) pain ladder

Pain does need treatment (pharmacological and non-pharmacological) and with this comes some guidance on side or unwanted effects that the prescriber or administering healthcare professional ought to know to inform the patient. There are cautions to be observed and discussed with patients needing pain relief. Patients taking prescribed medications may inadvertently take too much of a product causing overdosage if taking additional analgesia purchased OTC. Examples include cold and influenza (flu) preparations which contain paracetamol whilst already taking medications which contain paracetamol. Due to this the Government issues warnings and updates especially on labelling, guidance and also literature within medication packets (patient information leaflets) specifying warnings and duration of use. In 2020 MHRA (2020b) published further guidance updated from the 2014 guidance warning of the risks of addiction with OTC pain relief products containing codeine. This included improving advice and prompts for healthcare professionals when caring for and prescribing pain relief to patients. Healthcare professionals ought to also be aware of wider lifestyle or occupational aspects and the legal responsibilities with powerful analgesic medication. In March 2015 a new 'drug driving' law came into force (DoT, 2013) following a review of drugs and driving ability. This law makes it an offence to drive with certain drugs or prescription medicines above specified limits in the body which includes prescription drugs and specific non-prescription drugs (there is a 'zero tolerance' of so-called illegal drugs). The medicines covered by the law include sedatives such as diazepam but also analgesia including morphine. Since codeine is converted into morphine by the liver, it is included in the law, which means it may be an offence to drive while taking codeine.

Whilst a patient may feel in control, the reality is these drugs are powerful and will impair judgement to some degree.

Neuropathic pain deserves mentioning due to its complexity. It is often described as a 'shooting', 'burning', 'tingling' or 'numbness' sensation in a limb or other part of the body. Causes of neuropathic pain are complex and diverse. It has been proposed that is it associated with sensory nervous system impulses (Finnerup et al, 2020; Cheng, 2021) and may be attributed to damage (severing of the nerves or amputation), injury (compression), deterioration (diabetes neuropathy, myeloma), infection (syphilis) or spinal surgery. Since it is not possible to completely cure the underlying disease or lesion or to reverse the neurological changes, neuropathic pain is usually persistent.

Some pains have different treatment approaches, for example headache or migraine. Most headaches are time limited, i.e. last between 30 minutes and several hours and then resolve on their own and are not a sign of something more serious. The NHS (2021) advice is that if headaches persist and/or are accompanied by other features (nausea, vomiting, neck stiffness, fever etc.) then the headache is a sign of another pathology such as influenza or stroke. Migraines and cluster headaches are types of headaches which have a specific expression such as being located on one side of the head, throbbing and may be preceded by an 'aura' (sensory changes). The dominant 'headache' symptom is pain, however it is notable that the subjective experiences, mechanisms and causes may be very variable. Management of 'headache' of whatever type is often via simple analgesia (paracetamol or ibuprofen), but may require more specific prescribed medication.

GO FURTHER

Pain is complex – careful assessment is needed and consideration of altering/ lowering doses or ceasing medications may also be necessary. Not all pain can be treated with drugs and this ought to be considered holistically with care approaches. Read this revised definition of pain by the IASP and reflect on your own experiences, your patients and how you plan care for these patients' pharmacological and non-pharmacological approaches: www.iasp-pain.org/publications/iasp-news/ iasp-announces-revised-definition-of-pain/

Non-pharmacological approaches

A variety of non-pharmacological pain relief methods are available to relieve a patient's pain in a healthcare setting. These are used alongside pharmacological approaches but not as an alternative. Many non-pharmacological approaches trigger a relaxation response (stimulating the parasympathetic nervous system), but not all. In the main the action of some of these approaches is unknown, however they still do have a place within pain management. This will not be addressed here; readers are recommended to visit reputable texts to extend their knowledge on this.

GO FURTHER

Sometimes pain relief (analgesia) can cause problems in long-term use. Two such examples are:

- Headaches due to overuse of medication. This has been known to occur in people overusing simple pain medications or migraine medications (i.e. for more than 15 days per month) which impacts quality of life, functioning and leads to a cycle of stress and more headache pain. This requires careful management and review (NICE, 2022). The exact mechanism of this 'analgesia overuse' headache is unclear but thought to be a complex interaction of medication overuse and susceptibility.

  Suggested reading: https://cks.nice.org.uk/topics/headache-medication-overuse/

- Opioids: tolerance (i.e. needing higher doses for the same effect), dependency (physical and psychological need) and hyperalgesia (i.e. abnormal heightened pain sensitivity).

Suggested reading:

Opioid Aware: www.fpm.ac.uk/opioids-aware
Non pharmacological approaches to pain relief resources:

- Chronic pain NICE guideline [NG193] https://www.nice.org.uk/guidance/NG193
- Scottish Intercollegiate Guidelines Network (SIGN). (2019) Management of chronic pain, Quick Reference Guide. (SIGN no. 136). Edinburgh Available at: www.sign.ac.uk/our-guidelines/management-of-chronic-pain/
- Older adults: Pickering G, Zwakhalen S and Kaasalainen S (2018) Pain management in older adults: a nursing perspective. Cham: Springer.

The medicines list

- Non-opioids
- Non-steroidal anti-inflammatory medications (NSAIDs)
- Adjuvant drugs
- Weak opioids
- Strong opioids
- Compound preparations
- Neuropathic pain medications
- Specific headache (migraine/cluster headache) treatment

DRUG GROUPS/CONCEPT: NON-OPIOIDS AND NSAIDs

Non-opioids are a small group. However often combined with NSAIDS ensure a larger analgesic resource. The key non opioid here is paracetamol which is a familiar medication to many people. It is well known for its antipyretic (fever reducing) and analgesic properties. The exact mechanisms of action remains unclear but is possibly a consequence of weak inhibition of prostaglandins (PGs) synthesis or synthesis of COX-2 or 3 (see NSAIDS below) without the anti-inflammatory effect (Graham et al., 2013). Overall the mechanism is undetermined but this does not detract from its usefulness and importance in pain management.

Drug name: Paracetamol

UK brand names: Paramol

Average doses:

- Orally: 0.5-1 g every 4-6 hours; maximum 4 g per day

Intravenous infusion:

- Adults under 50 kg body weight: 15 mg/kg every 4-6 hours, administered over 15 minutes; maximum 60 mg/kg per day
- Adults over 50 kg body weight: 1 g every 4-6 hours, dose to be administered over 15 minutes; maximum 4 g per day

What form does it come in: Tablet, effervescent tablet, orodispersible tablet, capsule, oral suspension/solution, solution for infusion, suppository, powder

Does it interact with other medicines: Yes, the following interactions are known:

- Alcohol: in those who drink heavily, causes severe liver damage.
- Bedaquiline (for tuberculosis) - causes increased hepatic toxicity.
- Phenindione (anticoagulant) - increase the anticoagulant effect.

Non-steroidal anti-inflammatory medications (NSAIDs) treat both pain and inflammation. Inflammation is a contributing factor in many conditions, for example arthritis, back and neck pain conditions, so reducing inflammation often helps alleviate the pain. In regular full dosage NSAIDs have both a lasting analgesic and an anti-inflammatory effect which makes them particularly useful for the treatment of continuous or regular pain associated with inflammation (JFC, 2022). NSAIDs reduce the production of pain-causing chemicals in the body called 'prostaglandins'. These are produced by action of a family of enzymes: cyclo-oxygenase (COX) often labelled COX1, COX2 etc. NSAIDs vary in their selectivity for inhibiting different types of cyclo-oxygenase; selective inhibition of cyclo-oxygenase-2 (COX-2) is associated with less gastro-intestinal (GI) intolerance. The risk of GI bleeding, ulceration or perforation is higher with increasing NSAID doses, in patients with a history of ulcers, particularly if complicated with haemorrhage or perforation and in the elderly. Some NSAIDs have a higher risk of GI problems than others. This information drives drug selection for the individual patient.

Most common types of NSAIDs

There are many types of prescription and non-prescription (over-the-counter) NSAIDs. Although NSAIDs are commonly used, they are not suitable for everyone and can sometimes cause troubling side effects. NSAIDs should not be mixed, i.e. taking two from the group simultaneously, as this may impede their effectiveness. As always if in doubt ask the prescriber or pharmacist. The four NSAIDs most often used are:

- **Ibuprofen** is used to treat a wide range of inflammatory conditions including post-surgical pain and pain from inflammatory diseases, such as joint sprain and non-inflammatory conditions such as dysmenorrhea (menstrual pain) and influenza like symptoms. It is available in general sales over the counter and by prescription.
- **Aspirin** is less commonly used but can be used to treat pain, fever and inflammation. Low dose aspirin may also be used to reduce the risk of a thrombosis or myocardial infarction ('heart attack'). It is also available over the counter and sometimes by prescription.
- **Naproxen** is commonly used to treat pain from strained muscles, lower back pain, gout or dysmenorrhoea. It is available by prescription only in the UK.
- **Diclofenac** – similarly to the others, it treats pain and inflammation from a wide range of sources already mentioned but may also be used for migraine, toothache, joint sprain/strain. Oral tablets available on prescription only in the UK.
- **Celecoxib** (Celebrex). Celecoxib is a COX-2 inhibitor and most often used to treat pain caused by different forms of arthritis, including spinal osteoarthritis and rheumatoid arthritis. It is available on prescription only in the UK.

Other forms of NSAIDs

In addition to the above other NSAIDs are used in specific circumstances:

- **Ketorolac** can be given as an intravenous, intramuscular or intranasal drug, making it useful after surgery or if the patient cannot eat.
- **Indomethacin** – capsules and suppositories for rheumatic disease, other musculoskeletal disorders and dysmenorrhoea.
- **Mefenamic acid** – oral for dysmenorrhoea or menorrhagia (menstrual pain or heavy bleeding).

Drug group: Non-steroidal anti-inflammatory drugs (NSAIDs)

Drug name: Ibuprofen

UK brand names: Brufen, Ibuleve, Nurofen, Fenbid, Flarin

Average doses:

- 200–400 mg, 3-4 times a day; increased if needed up to a maximum of 600 mg four times a day. The daily maximum is 2.4 g

(Continued)

What form does it come in: Tablet, capsule, suspension, orodispersible, gastro-resistant tablet, modified release or topical gel

Does it interact with other medicines: Yes, the following interactions are known:

- Drugs which impair clotting, e.g. bemiparin, altaplace – antithrombotic drug, apixaban (impeded coagulation cascade).
- Beclometasone – increased risk of gastric bleeding if both taken.
- Dexomethasone, fludocortisone, methylprednisolone – increased risk of gastric bleeding if both taken.
- Dulexitine, escitalopram – serotonin-norepinephrine reuptake inhibitors used to treat depression and mental health conditions.
- Lithium – ibuprofen increases blood levels of lithium leading to potential toxicity.
- Zidovuzine – antiretroviral used for people with HIV. Increased risk of haematological toxicity.

Caution is recommended in patients with allergic disorders taking ibuprofen (and other NSAIDs) since this may worsen the allergeric response; cardiac impairment since NSAIDs may impair renal function; cerebrovascular disease due to potential vasoconstriction effects; coagulation defects due NSAID coagulation alterations; dehydration due to risk of renal impairment; elderly due to risk of serious side effects; and history of gastro-intestinal disorders (e.g. ulcerative colitis, Crohn's disease) due to the gastric irritating effects.

Drug name: Aspirin

UK brand names: Anadin, Disprin

Average doses:

- For mild pain: 300–900 mg every 4-6 hours as required; maximum 4 g per day
- Acute migraine: 900 mg for 1 dose as soon as migraine symptoms develop
- Cardiovascular disease, preventative (secondary) – 75 mg/day

What form does it come in: Tablet, dispersible tablet, gastro-resistant tablet, suppository

Does it interact with other medicines: Yes, there are several interactions some of which are known:

- Acetazolamide: used in glaucoma – increases the risk of severe toxic reaction.
- Oral antacids: impair absorption of aspirin.
- Other NSAIDs: diclofenac, dexketoprofen.
- Anti-clotting drugs, e.g. edoxaban: increases risk of bleeding.
- Fludrocortisone, beclomethasone (as for ibuprofen): increase risk of GI bleeding.

- Zidovuzine – antiretroviral used for people with HIV. Increased risk of haematological toxicity.

Caution for aspirin: adult patients with allergic disease due to increased potential for aspiring allergy; anaemia due to the altered coagulation and potential for bleeding; asthma due to potential increased sensitivity to aspirin; may mask symptoms of infection; previous peptic ulceration due to gastric irritation; and children due to risk of rare condition called Reyes syndrome.

Drug name: Naproxen

UK brand names: Naprosyn

Average doses:

- 0.5–1 g per days in 1–2 divided doses.

What form does it come in: Tablet, effervescent tablet, gastro-resistant tablet, oral suspension

Does it interact with other medicines: Yes, the following interactions are known:

- Same as ibuprofen and aspirin.

Caution: same as ibuprofen.

Drug name: Diclofenac

UK brand names: Voltarol, Dicloflex, Fenactol, Motifene

Average doses:

- 75–150 mg mg per day, in two or three divided doses.

What form does it come in: Tablet, gastro-resistant tablet, modified release capsules, topical gel (1.16% or 2.32%), medicated plasters, suppositories.

Does it interact with other medicines: Yes, The British National Formulary (JFC, 2022) cites 206 interactions some of which are very serious and need consideration for prescribing. The following key interactions are known and are route dependent:

(Continued)

- All NSAIDs and anticoagulants and anti-platelet agents with potential for increased risk of bleeding (gastrointestinal via oral route). Very serious.
- Selective serotonin reuptake inhibitors (SSRIs) – increased risk of GI bleeding.
- Zidovudine – increased risk of bleeding.
- Causes increased level of the following and potential toxicity:
  o Lithium
  o Methotrexate
  o Phenytoin
  o Mifepristone
  o Drugs which cause hyperkalaemia, e.g. ciclosporins, trimethoprim.
- Colestipol and cholestyramine – decreased metabolism of diclofenac.
- Diuretics and anti-hypertensive agents.
- Cardiac glycosides, e.g. digoxin. Diclofenac causes raised blood levels of digoxin, reduce glomerular filtration (excretion) and increase risk of cardiac failure.

Caution: In people with active gastro-intestinal bleeding as indicated above; active gastro-intestinal ulceration with risk of bleeding; history of gastro-intestinal bleeding related to previous NSAID therapy; cerebrovascular disease or ischaemic heart disease or mild to severe heart failure or peripheral arterial disease due to the concerns over COX-2 inhibitors and identified arterial thrombitic risks in this group of patients (MHRA, 2015).

Drug name: Celecoxib

UK brand names: Celebrex

Average doses:

- 200 mg per day in 1–2 divided doses

What form does it come in: Capsules

Does it interact with other medicines: Yes, the known interactions are the same as for diclofenac (see above).

Caution: Cardiovascular (CV) risks of celecoxib may increase with dose and duration of exposure thus it is recommended to use for the shortest duration possible and at the lowest effective daily dose, and reviewed frequently.

Drug name: Ketorolac

UK brand names: Acular, Toradol

Average doses:

- 10 mg initially, then 10 to 30mg every four to six hours as required (intramuscular or intravenously); eye drops (0.5%) – 1 drop four times a day post-surgery

What form does it come in: Solution for injection, eye drops

Does it interact with other medicines: Yes, the BNF cites 199 interactions and they are dependent on route (systemic versus topical eye drops). The interactions are as for diclofenac (above). In addition:

- Trometamol is not be administered alongside ketorolac therapy due to severe interaction (bleeding etc.).
- Probenecid – decreases elimination of ketorolac.

Caution: This is a short-term analgesia post-surgery. The cautions are the same as diclofenac but other people to consider include those with hepatic or renal insufficiency due to altered drug pharamockinetics, cardiac problems and hypertension (thrombotic risks), and pregnant women (crossing placenta).

Drug name: Indomethacin

UK brand names: Indocid

Average doses:

- 50-200 mg per day in 2 or 3 divided doses

What form does it come in: Capsules, suppositories

Does it interact with other medicines: Yes, the same as for diclofenac, plus the following interactions are known:

- Antidiabetic, i.e. sulfonylureas (glicazide, tolbutamide) due to raised levels by NSAIDs.
- Haloperidol (antipsychotic) results in increased levels and drowsiness.
- Antacids impair gastric absorption of indomethacin.
- Desmopressin may be potentiated or action increased.
- Baclofen (muscle relaxant) excretion decreased.

Drug name: Mefanamic acid

UK brand names: Ponstan

(Continued)

Average doses:

- 500 mg per day in three divided doses

What form does it come in: Capsules, oral suspension, film coated tablets

Does it interact with other medicines: Yes, the same as for diclofenac.

Caution when using with the elderly as the adverse effects may be severe, also in people with liver or renal failure due to potential altered metabolism and clearance. There is some suggestion it may impair female fertility and is not recommended in women attempting to conceive.

DRUG GROUP/CONCEPT: WEAK OPIOIDS AND STRONG OPIOIDS AND COMPOUND ANALGESIC PREPARATIONS

Opioid analgesics are an essential tool for some patients to manage pain and/or the healing process such as post-surgery. They have significant adverse effects and can lead to complications like delayed healing, tolerance or in extreme cases dependency. Their use is advocated for a limited time for these reasons, or as part of a holistic multimodal approach to pain management. Opioid drugs interact with naturally occurring receptors in the body termed 'opioid receptors'. This drug-receptor process produces pain relief at the spinal and central nervous system (CNS) (brain) level. These substances mimic the action of naturally occurring peptides collectively termed endogenous opioids or enkephalins. Their pharmacological actions on cells account for some of the other (or adverse) effects too – the reader is recommended to visit a good pharmacological textbook to elaborate on this. Suffice it to say an agonist such as morphine blocks the pain transmission and other transmission resulting in several side effects including respiratory depression and reduced gastrointestinal motility (constipation).

Examples of opioids (or weak opioids) for moderate pain include codeine, dihydrocodeine, tramadol and low dose oxycodone. These are used when pain is not relieved by non-opioid products and can often be found in compound formulations, e.g. co-codamol (paracetamol and codeine). If these medications are ineffective the next type of opioids would be those recommended for moderate to severe pain (strong opioids), including: morphine, oxycodone, fentanyl, diamorphine and hydromorphone. Opioids are available in a variety of formulations and can be administered through a variety of routes, the most common being oral, subcutaneous and intravenous. Oral opioids are available in both short-acting and long-acting (modified, controlled or extended release) forms. Intravenous patient controlled analgesia allows patients to manage their own pain by self-administering opioid doses and is one of the most commonly used methods to treat acute pain post-operatively. Other routes for opioid use are epidural or intrathecal.

Compound analgesic preparations contain a simple analgesic (such as aspirin or paracetamol) with an opioid in a relatively small dose in the management of short-term pain of varying intensity. All the elements have an active ingredient which theoretically may complement or add to the action of the other. The role of these in pain management is not well documented (JFC, 2022) and in the main the presence of an opioid makes them a concern for adverse events even in small doses. Furthermore, the presence of two drugs complicates the management if there was any overdose. Because of concerns about safety and the risk of abuse, the legislation around these drugs is tight and OTC packets of these drugs are limited to 32 tablets; anything over this is prescription only. Generally daily maximum doses are limited by the safety of the simple analgesic, i.e. paracetamol. There are five types of compound analgesics containing paracetamol, and only one with aspirin (Chaplin and Campbell, 2014):

- Co-codaprin (aspirin 400 mg, codeine 8 mg)
- Co-codamol 8/500 (paracetamol 500 mg, codeine 8 mg)
- Co-codamol 15/500 (paracetamol 500 mg, codeine 15 mg)
- Co-codamol 30/500 (paracetamol 500 mg, codeine 30 mg)
- Co-dydramol (paracetamol 500 mg with either 10 mg, 20 mg or 30 mg dihydrocodeine)
- Paracetamol and tramadol (paracetamol 325 mg, tramadol 37.5 mg)

Drug groups/concept: Compound analgesic preparations

Drug name: Aspirin and codeine combination product

UK brand names: Co-codaprin

Average doses:

- Aspirin 400 mg, codeine 8 mg: 1-2 tablets every 4-6 hours as required; maximum 8 tablets per day

What form does it come in: Dispersible tablets

Does it interact with other medicines: Yes, see interactions for aspirin and interactions for codeine.

Caution: Not suitable for prescribing - OTC limited to 32 tablets.

Drug name: Paracetamol and codeine combination product

UK brand names: Co-codamol, Solpadol, Kapake

Average doses:

- 8/500 mg: 1-2 tablets every 4-6 hours as required; maximum 64/4000 mg per day (8 tablets)

(Continued)

- 15/500 mg: 1-2 tablets every 4-6 hours as required; maximum 120/4000 mg per day (8 tablets)
- 30/500 mg: 1-2 tablets every 4-6 hours as required; maximum 240/4000 mg per day (8 tablets)

What form does it come in: Capsules, caplets, effervescent tablets

Does it interact with other medicines: Yes, see interactions for aspirin and interactions for codeine.

Caution: MHRA reminds healthcare professionals that opioids co-prescribed with benzodiazepines and benzodiazepine-like drugs can produce additive CNS depressant effects, thereby increasing the risk of sedation, respiratory depression, coma and death (JFC, 2022). Drowsiness impedes driving, operating machinery or high-risk activities. Not for use during pregnancy or whilst breastfeeding.

Drug name: Tramadol with paracetamol (37.5 mg/325 mg)

UK brand names: Tramacet

Average doses:

- 37.5 mg/325 mg: 1-2 tablets every 6 hours not exceeding 8 tablets/day

What form does it come in: Tablets, effervescent tablets

Does it interact with other medicines: Yes, see interactions for paracetamol and interactions for tramadol.

Drug name: Dihydrocodeine and paracetamol

UK brand names: Eroset, Paramol, Remedeine Forte

Average doses:

- 10/500 mg: 1-2 tablets every 4-6 hours as required; maximum 80/4000 mg per day (8 tablets)
- 20/500 mg: 1-2 tablets every 4-6 hours as required; maximum 160/4000 mg per day (8 tablets)
- 30/500 mg: 1-2 tablets every 4-6 hours as required; maximum 240/4000 mg per day (8 tablets)

What form does it come in: Tablets

Does it interact with other medicines: Yes, see interactions for paracetamol and interactions for dihydrocodeine.

Drug groups/concept: Opioids

Drug name: Codeine

UK brand names: None

Average doses:

- Pain: 30-60 mg every 4 hours as required; maximum 240 mg per day
- Acute diarrhoea: 30 mg, 3-4 times a day
- Cough: 15-30 mg, 3-4 times a day

What form does it come in: Tablet, linctus and oral solution

Does it interact with other medicines: Yes, the BNF states over 126 drug interactions. The following interactions are known:

- Alcohol - hypotensive, sedative and respiratory depressive effects of alcohol may be enhanced.
- Mexiletine (antiarrhythmic) absorption reduced.
- Enhanced sedative effects with drug types including:
  o Antihistamines
  o Antipsychotics
  o Antidepressants
  o Anxiolytics and hypnotics
  o Benzodiazepines.
- Cimetidine may inhibit the metabolism of codeine.

Caution: Pregnancy and breastfeeding due to passing through the placenta or breast milk to. Driving and operating machinery or extreme physical activities since these can cause drowsiness.

Drug name: Dihydrocodeine

UK brand names: DF118 Forte

Average doses:

- 30 mg every 4-6 hours as required; maximum 180 mg per day (6 tablets)
- 60-120 mg every 12 hours (modified release)

What form does it come in: Tablet, modified release, oral solution

(Continued)

Does it interact with other medicines: Yes, the JFC (2022) states 120 drug interactions. The following interactions are known:

- Enhanced sedative effects with drug types including:
  - Anaesthetics
  - Antihistamines (sedating)
  - Antipsychotics (clozapine)
  - Antidepressants
  - Anxiolytics and hypnotics
  - Benzodiazepines
  - Antiemetics (cyclizine).
- Alcohol-enhanced hypotensive, sedative effect and respiratory depression.
- Mexiletine - absorption delayed.
- Cimetidine - inhibit the metabolism of opioids.

Caution: As for codeine.

Drug name: Tramadol

UK brand names: Maxitram, Brimisol, Zydol, Tilodol, Tramuleif

Average doses:

- 50-100 mg every 4-6 hours; maximum 400 mg per day
- 150-200 mg twice daily (modified release) maximum 400 mg per day

What form does it come in: Capsule, modified-release capsule, soluble tablet, dispersible tablet, modified-release tablet, oral solution, oral drops, solution for injection

Does it interact with other medicines: Yes, this includes all those within the codeine list, and the following additional interactions are known:

- Buprenorphine and pentazocine (partial agonist analgesia) reduces the effect of tramadol.
- Carbamazepine - reduces the effect of tramadol
- Selegiline (a mono amine oxidase inhibitor) and tricyclic antidepressants increase risk of serotonin syndrome, e.g. agitation, insomnia, confusion, hypertension, convulsions.
- Clozapine - enhanced risk of constipations with tramadol and potential for GI obstruction.

Drug name: Oxycodone

UK brand names: Onexila, Ixyldone, Lontec, Linlor

Average doses:

- Oral: 5 mg every 4-6 hours (titrated to pain level), maximum 400 mg per day
- Oral: 10 mg every 12 hours; maximum 400 mg per day (modified release)
- Subcutaneous injection: 5 mg every 4 hours
- Intravenous infusion: 2 mg/hour

What form does it come in: Tablet, modified-release tablet, capsule, oral solution, solution for injection

Does it interact with other medicines: Yes, this includes all those within the codeine list, and the following additional interactions are known:

- Rifampicin, carbamazepine, phenytoin and St John's Wort may induce liver enzymes to metabolise oxycodone (reduce the levels).
- Itraconazole, ketoconazole, paroxetine, ritonavir and quinidine – liver enzyme inhibitor causes increase in oxycodone levels.
- Grapefruit juice – inhibits liver enzymes and increases oxycodone levels.

Drug name: Morphine sulphate

UK brand names: Actimorph, Cylcimorph, Morphgesic, MST, MSL, Sevredol

Average doses: Dose adjusted according to the response (i.e. if it does not improve pain then increased dose):

- Acute pain (adults): 10 mg every 4 hours (oral, subcutaneous or intramuscular injection); or 5 mg every 4 hours (slow intravenous injection)
- Acute pain (elderly): 5 mg every 4 hours (oral, subcutaneous or intramuscular injection)
- Chronic pain (adults): 5-10 mg every 4 hours (oral, subcutaneous or intramuscular injection); or 15-30 mg every 4 hours (rectal suppository)
- Modified release pain relief (adults): dose adjusted according to daily morphine requirements with modified-release 12-hourly preparations (i.e. twice a day)

What form does it come in: Tablet, orodispersible tablet, modified-release tablet, modified-release capsule, oral solution, solution for injection, solution for infusion

(Continued)

Does it interact with other medicines: Yes, the JFC (2022) states 122 drug interactions. The following known interactions are some of these:

- Alcohol: enhance the pharmacodynamic effects (CNS depressant) causing enhanced adverse effects and may be life threatening.
- Monoamine oxidase inhibitors (isocarboxazid, phenelzine sulphate, tranylcypromine) via increased stimulant (serotonin syndrome).
- Cimetidine – inhibits metabolism of morphine.
- CNS depressants: amitriptyline, phenothiazine and other sedative medicines such as benzodiazepines increases the risk of sedation, respiratory depression, coma and death (additive CNS depressant effect).
- Mixed agonist/antagonist opioid analgesics (e.g. buprenorphine, nalbuphine, pentazocine) – conflicting effects (opioid withdrawal).
- Clozapine: intestinal obstruction due to enhanced constipating effect.

Caution: A person's judgement and dexterity skills may be severely affected. There is also a risk of dependence and addiction (MHRA, 2020a). Morphine readily crosses the placenta and into breast milk. In the control of pain in terminal illness, the cautions listed should not necessarily be a deterrent to the use of opioid analgesics and doses may be higher. Caution is also advised when changing routes, e.g. the dose for oral administration is not the same for intramuscular – this is for the person administering the drug to be aware of and the prescriber to confirm referring to a clinical conversion algorithm.

Drug name: Fentanyl

UK brand names: Actiq, Abstral, Instanyl, Cinril, Efentora, PecFent

Average doses (caution if also taking other opioids):

- Chronic intractable pain: Transdermal patch: 12 to 25 micrograms/hour every 72 hours. Evaluation of the dose analgesic effect at a minimum of 24 hours
- Breakthrough pain in patients receiving opioid therapy:
  o Buccal lozenges: 200 micrograms, dose to be given over 15 minutes, then 200 micrograms after 15 minutes if required, no more than 2 dose units for each pain episode
  o Buccal film: 200 micrograms, adjusted according to response, consult product literature for information on dose adjustments, maximum 1.2 mg per episode of breakthrough pain

    o   Sublingual tablets: 100 micrograms, then 100 micrograms after 15-30 minutes if required, maximum of 800 micrograms per episode of breakthrough pain

    o   Intranasal spray: 50 micrograms, dose to be administered into one nostril, then 50 micrograms after 10 minutes if required, maximum 2 sprays for each pain episode

What form does it come in: Sublingual tablet, buccal tablet, buccal film, lozenge, solution for injection, solution for infusion, transdermal patch, nasal spray

Does it interact with other medicines: Yes, the JFC (2022) states 230 drug interactions. The following severe interactions are known:

- Same as for opioids.
- CNS depressants, such as other morphine derivatives (analgesics and antitussives), general anaesthetics, gabapentinoids (gabapentin and pregabalin), skeletal muscle relaxants, sedative antidepressants, sedative antihistamines, barbiturates, anxiolytics (i.e. benzodiazepines), hypnotics, antipsychotics, clonidine, and related substances may produce increased CNS depressant effects, increased risk of sedation, respiratory depression, hypotension, coma and death because of additive CNS depressant effect.
- Atazanavir, darunavir, fosamprenavir (HIV drugs): increase effect of fentanyl.
- Ketoconazole, vorizonazole: increases effect of fentanyl.

Drug name: Diamorphine

Other UK brand names: None

Average doses:

- Acute pain: 5 mg every 4 hours (intramuscular injection or subcutaneous injection)
- Chronic pain: 2.5-5 mg every 4 hours (intramuscular injection or subcutaneous injection)

What form does it come in: Powder for solution (injection ampoules)

Does it interact with other medicines: Yes, the JFC (2022) states 230 drug interactions, including the following known interactions:

- Same as for opioids.
- Alcohol: effects enhanced.
- Mexitiline (antiarrhythmic).
- Antidiarrhoeal and antiperistaltic agents (such as loperamide and kaolin): simultaneous use increases severe constipation.

(Continued)

Drug name: Hydromorphone

UK brand names: Palladone, Palladone SR

Average doses:

- Capsules: 1.3 mg every 4 hours, increasing dose if necessary according to severity of cancer pain
- Modified release capsules: 4 mg every 12 hours, increasing dose if necessary according to severity of cancer pain

What form does it come in: Capsule, modified release capsule

Does it interact with other medicines: Yes, the following interactions are known:

- Same as for opioids.

Drug name: Gabapentin

UK brand names: Neurontin

Average doses: Scaled dose depending on the individual's response:

- 300 mg once daily
- Increased in steps of 300 mg every 2–3 days in 3 divided doses
- Maximum 3.6 g per day.

What form does it come in: Tablet, capsule, oral solution

Does it interact with other medicines: Yes, the following interactions are known:

- CNS depressants (e.g. alcohol, morphine, fentanyl, benzodiazepines) causing increased CNS depressant effects, increased risk of sedation, altered dexterity and coordination.

Caution: This drug is also used for other conditions, for example focal seizures.

Drug name: Pregabalin

UK brand names: Lyrica, Alzain, Axalid

Average doses: Scaled dose depending on the individual's response:

- 150 mg daily in 2-3 divided doses
- Then increased if necessary to 300 mg daily in 2-3 divided doses
- Then increased if necessary up to 600 mg daily in 2-3 divided doses

What form does it come in: Tablet, capsule, oral solution

Does it interact with other medicines: Yes, the following interactions are known:

- CNS depressants (e.g. alcohol, morphine, fentanyl, benzodiazepines) causing increased CNS depressant effects, increased risk of sedation, altered dexterity and coordination.

Caution: This drug is also used for other conditions, for example focal seizures.

Drug name: Capsaicin

UK brand names: Axsain, Qutenza, Zaicin

Average doses:

- 0.075% strength cream; applied sparingly 3-4 times a day, not more often than every 4 hours

What form does it come in: Cream, cutaneous patch

Does it interact with other medicines: No

Caution: Not for use on broken or irritated skin (e.g. herpetic lesions) due to irritant effect.

HEADACHES (MIGRAINE OR CLUSTER HEADACHES)

These expressions of pain require management either with more conservative approaches (rest, hydration, avoiding stress or triggers etc.) or with drug therapy. Simple analgesia such as paracetamol or ibuprofen early in the headache experience may be effective, however other treatments such as the triptan group of medications (serotonin 5HT1 receptor agonists) are advocated if pain worsens (SIGN, 2018).

Drug groups/concept: Triptan

Drug name: Sumatriptan

UK brand names: Imigran, Migraitan

Average doses:

- Oral: 50-100 mg for 1 dose, followed by 50-100 mg after at least 2 hours if required: maximum of 300 mg a day
- Subcutaneous injection: 3-6 mg for 1 dose, followed by 3-6 mg after at least 1 hour if required. Maximum 12 mg a day
- Intranasal spray: 10-20 mg, to be administered into one nostril, followed by 10-20 mg after at least 2 hours if required. Maximum 40 mg a day

What form does it come in: Tablet, solution for injection, nasal spray

Does it interact with other medicines: Yes, the following interactions are known:

- Drugs which alter serotonin levels such as antiemetics (HT receptor agonists) or antidepressant medication: SSRIs, serotonin and norepinephrine reuptake inhibitors, or mono amine oxidase inhibitors:
  - Bupropion: enhances risk of serotonin syndrome
  - Ergotamine: risk of vasoconstriction (myocardial or cerebral blood flow impairment)
  - Isocarboxazid: enhances levels of sumatriptan
  - Ondansetron: enhances risk of serotonin syndrome
  - Granisetron: enhances risk of serotonin syndrome
  - St Johns Wort: enhances risk of serotonin syndrome
  - Opioids (tramadol, tapentadol): enhances risk of serotonin syndrome.

Caution: When using in people with cardiovascular conditions, hypertension or seizures due to the powerful vaso-constrictive actions of these medications.

GO FURTHER

Medication overuse headache (MOH) is a type of headache that develops and gets worse with frequent use of any medication treatment. People who have tension-type headaches or migraines and take analgesia such as triptans, ergotamines, opiates, NSAIDs and paracetamol are susceptible to MOH. It develops in people with a primary headache disorder, such as migraine (or a family history of migraine), usually with a headache on 15 or more days per month. The medicine itself causes more headaches, which are sometimes referred to as 'rebound headaches'.

Read more here: https://cks.nice.org.uk/topics/headache-medication-overuse/

ANALGESIA IN PREGNANCY AND BREASTFEEDING

Various kinds of pain may occur (headaches, backache or other pain) during pregnancy. In the main drugs ought to be avoided during pregnancy to avoid harm to the developing foetus (MHRA, 2021). If clinically required, paracetamol may be taken, however it is recommended to be of the lowest effective dose for the shortest possible time and at the lowest possible frequency. Paracetamol is excreted in breast milk but not in a significant amount. Furthermore, while no teratogenic (foetus damaging) effects have been demonstrated with use of ibuprofen, if possible, it should be avoided during the first six months of pregnancy. During the third trimester (12 weeks), ibuprofen is to be avoided completely as there is a risk of premature closure of the foetal ductus arteriosus with possible persistent cardiac issues and pulmonary hypertension. Also the onset of labour may be delayed and duration of labour increased with ibuprofen (JFC, 2022). It may appear in breast milk, and several manufacturers and the MHRA (2021) advise avoiding ibuprofen and NSAIDs whilst breastfeeding. Given the powerful effect of combination drugs and opioids these are to be avoided as they may cause respiratory depression and withdrawal symptoms in the neonate. These drugs also cross through breast milk and so it is recommended they be avoided.

CAUTIONS WITH ANALGESIA

These have been outlined within the differing drug summary monographs above. All drugs have effects, adverse effects and toxicity concerns. Analgesia is particularly concerning as drugs such as paracetamol and ibuprofen are readily available over the counter (also see Chapter 8) and may be viewed as mild and not dangerous or inadvertently taken to excess. Most people are aware that opioids are dangerous and a key concern is tolerance, addiction or withdrawal effects in individuals taking them when managing pain or medication regimes.

LEARNING FROM A CASE STUDY:
TEST YOUR KNOWLEDGE

Oscar is a 38-year-old with chronic lower back and leg pain. Three years ago, Oscar was involved in a serious motorcycle incident resulting in orthopaedic surgery for various fractures. Back pain developed then and has remained unresolved, for which oxycodone is prescribed (when needed/*pro re nata*). It is time to review the medication and Oscar wants to continue with the oxycodone in doses of 15 mg, five times a day. Oscar describes this as providing 'fair' pain relief. It appears the pain is worse at night and impacts on sleep causing worry and stress around work and keeping their job.

1   Should this back pain be treated with opiates?
2   What might you ask about the timing between doses? Are there options?
3   Why do you think Oscar is only experiencing 'fair' pain relief with the current dose of oxycodone?
4   What do Oscar's reports on sleep and thoughts about work point to?

IF I REMEMBER 5 THINGS FROM THIS CHAPTER:

1 Pain is a complex sensation and is unique to the person experiencing it.
2 Pain can be treated with a holistic approach which includes pharmacological and non-pharmacological means.
3 Treatment starts with the lowest dose of the weakest analgesia titrating (scaling) up according to the individual's response to the medication.
4 Even the simplest analgesics have serious adverse effects, for example paracetamol can impair liver enzymes and lead to irreparable damage, or NSAIDs amend to 'can cause' gastrointestinal irritation.
5 Stronger analgesics have multiple interactions with other drugs including alcohol and caution is needed to minimise the adverse risks and very serious consequences.

ANSWERS TO CASE STUDY QUESTIONS

1 Opioids are very powerful drugs and are used for short-term acute conditions such as back pain after injury. They are not recommended for long-term chronic problems due to their adverse effects and risks of tolerance, dependency and also for the potential for a rebound effect of increased pain sensitivity.
2 It may be the timing means the blood level of the drugs and thus pain relief are ineffective. It may be that the short-term action of oxycodone is offering peaks of pain relief and not consistent pain relief so a longer acting preparation may be appropriate.
3 Over a long period of time and taking the stated dose still shows signs of being tolerant to the drug. It may be that a review of lifestyle, non-drug means or another opiate compound with a different structure may be more effective.
4 Stress and anxiety can aggravate and intensify pain sensation. It may be that Oscar has other worries which may need referral, for example to wellbeing or counselling services or even to assess for depression. Stress can exacerbate pain, and pain can also exacerbate stress. Adjuvants such as antidepressants may assist in the management of pain too.

REFERENCES AND RECOMMENDED READING

Chaplin, S. and Campbell, W. (2014) Properties and use of compound analgesics in pain management. *Prescriber, 24*(1–2): 38–40. https://doi.org/10.1002/psb.1006

Cheng, J. (2021) Is It Time to Redefine Neuropathic Pain? *Pain Medicine, 22* (12): 2801–2802. Available at: https://doi.org/10.1093/pm/pnab168

Department of Transport (DoT) (2013) Changes to drug driving law – Road Traffic Act. Available at: www.gov.uk/government/collections/drug-driving

Finnerup, N. R., Kuner, R., Jensen, T. S. (2020) Neuropathic Pain: From Mechanisms to Treatment. *Physiological Reviews*, 101: 259–301. Available at: https://doi.org/10.1152/physrev.00045.2019

Graham, G.G., Davies, M.J., Day, R.O., Mohamudally, A., Scott, K.F. (2013) The modern pharmacology of paracetamol: therapeutic actions, mechanism of action, metabolism, toxicity and recent pharmacological findings. *Inflammopharmacology*, *21*(3):201–32. doi: 10.1007/s10787-013-0172-x.

International Association for the Study of Pain (IASP) (2022) News alert: IASP announces revised definition of pain. Available at: www.iasp-pain.org/publications/iasp-news/iasp-announces-revised-definition-of-pain/

Joint Formulary Committee (JFC) (2022) *British National Formulary*. London: BMJ and Pharmaceutical Press. Available at: https://bnf.nice.org.uk/

Medicines and Healthcare Products Regulatory Agency (MHRA) (2020a) Press release: UK regulator strengthens opioid warnings. Available at: www.gov.uk/government/news/uk-regulator-strengthens-opioid-warnings

Medicines and Healthcare Products Regulatory Agency (MHRA) (2020b) Opioid medicines and the risk of addiction. Safety leaflet. Available at: www.gov.uk/guidance/opioid-medicines-and-the-risk-of-addiction

Medicines and Healthcare Regulatory Authority (2015) Guidance Cox-2 selective inhibitors and non-steroidal anti-inflammatory drugs (NSAIDs): Cardiovascular safety. Available at: https://www.gov.uk/government/publications/cox-2-selective-inhibitors-and-non-steroidal-anti-inflammatory-drugs-nsaids-cardiovascular-safety/cox-2-selective-inhibitors-and-non-steroidal-anti-inflammatory-drugs-nsaids-cardiovascular-safety

Medicines and Healthcare Regulatory Authority (2021) Guidance: Use of medicines in pregnancy and breastfeeding. Available at: https://www.gov.uk/guidance/use-of-medicines-in-pregnancy-and-breastfeeding

National Institute for Health and Care Excellence (NICE) (2019) Clinical knowledge summaries: Neuropathic pain – drug treatment. Available at: https://cks.nice.org.uk/topics/neuropathic-pain-drug-treatment/

National Institute for Health and Care Excellence (2021) Analgesia – mild-to-moderate pain. Clinical Knowledge Summaries. Available at: https://cks.nice.org.uk/topics/analgesia-mild-to-moderate-pain/

National Institute for Health and Care Excellence (NICE) (2022) Clinical knowledge summaries: Headache – assessment. Available at: https://cks.nice.org.uk/topics/headache-assessment/

National Health Service (NHS) (2021) Health topics: Headaches. Available at: www.nhs.uk/conditions/headaches/

Raja, S.N., Carr, D.B., Cohen, M., Finnerup, N.B., Flor, H., Gibson, S., Keefe, F.J., Mogil, J.S., Ringkamp, M., Sluka, K.A., Song, X.J., Stevens, B., Sullivan, M.D., Tutelman, P.R., Ushida, T., Vader, K. (2020) The revised International Association for the Study of Pain definition of pain: concepts, challenges, and compromises. *Pain, 161*(9): 1976–1982. doi: 10.1097/j.pain.0000000000001939.

Scottish Intercollegiate Guidelines Network (SIGN) (2018) National clinical guideline 155: Pharmacological management of migraine. Available at: www.sign.ac.uk/our-guidelines/pharmacological-management-of-migraine/

World Health Organisation (1986) Cancer Pain Relief. Geneva, WHO. Available at: https://iris.who.int/bitstream/handle/10665/43944/9241561009_eng.pdf;jsessionid=B529EFB089 66EB8A37785FF6AB48CACE?sequence=1

8 MEDICINES FOR COMMON SYMPTOMS

SHEILA CUNNINGHAM

AFTER READING THIS CHAPTER YOU WILL BE ABLE TO:

- Describe common signs and symptoms.
- List at least one key medication for each symptom explored.
- Consider the risks and benefits of the medications for key symptoms and the role of self-care symptom relief.
- Apply knowledge to support clinical decision making.

OVERVIEW

Nurses learn the biological and pathological processes in disease development. Nurses also learn some conceptual basis to disease, i.e. pathophysiological response or alteration to tissues or organs and the terminology surrounding this such as 'disorder' or 'disease' labels. Examples include inflammation and degeneration in osteoarthritis or bacterial or viral growth and infection. Disorder in general refers to a functional abnormality or disturbance, e.g. endocrine disorder, whilst illness refers to the person's personal experience of the disease/disorder. Signs and symptoms are features aligned with disease and disorder processes and may be unique to that disease or disorder (e.g. growths) or broader. Signs in general refer to the objective features of a disease or disorder (swelling, tissue alteration) whereas symptoms are more qualitative and affective (e.g. pain, distress, nausea). There are times when symptoms are not due to pathologies but due to life stresses, vulnerabilities or behavioural choices, e.g. vulnerability to pollen (hayfever) or travel sickness. Many diseases and disorders have symptoms in common, hence 'common symptoms'. Drugs or medicines to alleviate symptoms exist and are available either with or without prescription, over the counter (OTC) at pharmacies or supermarkets.

The manufacture and supply of medicines are regulated under legislation which affects how and where you can obtain them. There are several key laws pertinent to medicines, but it is not within the scope of this chapter to address all of these, so it is recommended the reader visit a text such as the British National Formulary (JFC, 2023) or other literature. A review was undertaken in 2018 by NHS England partnered with NHS Clinical Commissioners (2018) and guidance was produced for GPs and prescribers on conditions for which they ought not to prescribe. The rationale was that since those illnesses are often self-limiting the medicines were a huge drain on limited NHS resources and either not needed or the patient could buy them themselves. Furthermore, the review indicated that medicines are often of limited clinic effectiveness; minor conditions such as sore throats, colds, mouth ulcers, sore rectums from diarrhoea or itchiness due to head lice are more suited to self-care to address symptoms. For these common conditions and symptoms OTC self-administered therapy may be recommended by the nurse or healthcare professional.

In 2019 NHS England and Clinical Commissioners published revised commissioning guidance on reducing prescribing of medicines which can be obtained OTC. In total there is a list of 35 conditions in this category, medicines for which one can buy OTC and will no longer be prescribed. There are exceptions to this such as for patients with long-term conditions, complex minor conditions, the inability to self-manage and others (BMA, 2019). This makes it more critical that when encountering patients, the healthcare professional needs to be very clear on what medicines they are taking, including self-administered OTC, any prescription medicines, increasingly any herbal medicines and any interactions and concerns which may arise.

Every OTC medicine has one or more specific 'active ingredients' that enable the medicine to act on tissues. For example, the active ingredient in cough and cold medicine could be paracetamol or pseudoephedrine which reduces fever or pain or relieves a cough. Needless to say, if symptoms are not improving, or patients are not responding to treatment or worsening, then they need to seek further advice. There are cautions. Medicines are licensed for particular use and the product licence may inhibit product sale OTC to certain groups of patients. This may vary by medicine, but community pharmacists are best placed to advise for groups such as babies, children and/or women who are pregnant or breastfeeding.

GO FURTHER

The Common Ailments Service initiative in Wales covers free treatment for 26 ailments: https://thepracticeofhealth.nhs.wales/clinics-services/self-help-care/minor-common-ailments/

This chapter will address a selection of medicines for the management of the following common symptoms (excluding children and babies).

COMMON SYMPTOMS ADDRESSED WITHIN THIS CHAPTER

- Acute sore throat
- Conjunctivitis
- Coughs, colds and nasal congestion
- Diarrhoea (adults)
- Haemorrhoids
- Indigestion and heartburn
- Infrequent migraine
- Vomiting (including motion or travel sickness)
- Mild or infrequent constipation
- Mild to moderate hayfever

COMMON SYMPTOMS ADDRESSED IN OTHER CHAPTERS

- Minor conditions associated with pain, discomfort and fever (e.g. aches and sprains, headache, period pain, back pain) – see Chapter 7
- Oral thrush – see Chapter 3
- Ringworm/athletes foot – see Chapter 3

SYMPTOM: ACUTE SORE THROAT

Acute sore throat is a common condition. In a survey study conducted in Scotland, 31% of adults reported a severe sore throat in the previous year, with 38% of these people seeking medical help (Kenealy, 2014). Also known as 'pharyngitis' it can be a sign of other ailments which ought to be explored so the appropriate treatment, if any, is chosen. For example, pharyngitis may be an indicator of a common cold (coryza), Group A streptococcal pharyngitis/tonsillitis, infectious mononucleosis (glandular fever) or measles (NICE, 2022). In the main a sore throat due to a viral or bacterial cause is a self-limiting condition. Symptoms often resolve within three days in 40% of people, and within one week in 85% of people, irrespective of whether or not the sore throat is due to a streptococcal infection (NICE, 2022). There is little evidence to suggest that treatments such as lozenges or throat sprays help to treat the cause of sore throat and patients should be advised to take simple painkillers and implement some self-care measures such as gargling with warm salty water instead.

If the pain from the sore throat is unbearable simple analgesia is a suggested option. This can be bought OTC in shops and pharmacies, e.g. paracetamol or ibuprofen. Details of these can be found in Chapter 7.

Drug group: Benzydamine

Drug name: Benzydamine

UK brand names: Difflam

Average doses:

- Rinse or gargle with 15 ml every 1.5 to 3 hours

What form does it come in: Sprays, mouthwash, gargle

Duration of therapy: Maximum of three days

Caution: Not advisable in patients with hypersensitivity to acetylsalicylic acid or other NSAIDs.

Does it interact with other medicines: No (topical)

SYMPTOM: COUGHS, COLDS AND NASAL CONGESTION

Most coughs and colds are short time-limited viral infections. On average adults get four to six colds per year, while children get six to eight of them (Barrett, 2018). There are more than 200 viruses, continuously changing, that are associated with the 'common cold' with coronaviruses generally associated with more severe symptoms than rhinoviruses (Barrett, 2018). Colds and influenza with the accompanying cough and nasal congestion occur in seasonal waves. Interestingly, post-Covid with more social integration there is increasing incidences of such viral infections which may or may not be associated with and worsened by Covid (PHE, 2022). Vaccines are available for seasonal influenza strains for vulnerable people, but colds and coughs are generally not vaccinated against due to the prolific range and evolution of cold viruses. In the main the minor viral respiratory ailments are self-limiting, if uncomfortable, and they often improve within 7–10 days; however at times coughs may take longer to clear up, i.e. within 2–3 weeks. Both of these conditions can result in nasal congestion and at times pain in the front of the head. Neither condition requires any treatment, though the symptoms may be uncomfortable and require some support. Coughing, however, may be a symptom of an underlying disorder such as asthma or gastro-oesophageal reflux disease, or a consequence of another medicine (NHS Inform, n.d.). This should be addressed before prescribing and will be guided by the pharmacist if OTC medication is obtained. Congestion may be treated with decongestants; most cold and influenza preparations contain a mild analgesia and decongestant.

Drug name: Pseudoephedrine hydrochloride

UK brand names: Sudafed, Galpseud, Lemsip (with paracetamol)

Average doses:

- 60 mg, 3-4 times a day

What form does it come in: Tablets and oral solution

Does it interact with other medicines: Yes, the following interactions are known:

- Isocarboxazid, moclobemide, phenelzine, tranylcypromine (for depression) - increases risk of hypertensive crisis.
- Linezolid (antibacterial) - increases risk of hypertension.
- Ozanimod (multiple sclerosis) - increases risk of hypertensive crisis.
- Rasagiline, safinamide, selegiline (Parkinson's disease) - increases risk of hypertensive crisis.

Caution: In people with heart disease; hypertension among others since this medicine can cause an increase in heart rate or blood pressure (stimulant action).

Drug name: Pholcodine

UK brand names: Covonia, Galenphol, Hill's Balsam

Average doses:

- 5-10 mg, 3-4 times a day

What form does it come in: Oral solution

Does it interact with other medicines: Yes, the following interactions are known:

- Isocarboxazid, moclobemide, phenelzine, tranylcypromine (for depression) - increases risk of nervous excitation or depression.

SYMPTOM: DIARRHOEA (ADULTS)

Diarrhoea is the abnormal passing of loose or liquid stools, with increased frequency, increased volume or both. It is a common symptom and can cause distress and embarrassment. It normally lasts a few days up to a week if it is a rare occurrence. It can be the consequence of a gastrointestinal infection (gastroenteritis either viral or bacterial), bacteria in contaminated food (*Campylobacter* and *Escherichia coli*), contaminated water (e.g. when travelling such as the parasite giardiasis), a food allergy, a side effect of a drug, or due to a chronic condition such as Crohn's disease, irritable bowel syndrome or ulcerative colitis. If it persists longer than a week then investigation is needed to eliminate more sinister causes and problems. However in the short term for acute diarrhoea the key aims are the prevention or reversal of fluid and electrolyte depletion and the management of dehydration with water and rehydration electrolyte supplements (JFC, 2023). There are medicines to slow or cease diarrhoea.

Drug group: Antimotility

Drug name: Loperamide hydrochloride

UK brand names: Imodium

Average doses:

- Initially 4 mg, followed by 2 mg for up to five days, dose to be taken after each loose stool; usual dose 6–8 mg daily; maximum 16 mg per day.

What form does it come in: Tablet, orodispersible tablet, capsule

Duration of therapy: Maximum up to five days

Does it interact with other medicines: Yes, the following serious interactions are known:

- Clozepine: both cause constipation enhancing the effect.
- Desmopressin - increased oral absorption of desmopressin.
- Dronedarone: increases effect of lopermide.
- Tepotinib: increases effect of lopermide.

SYMPTOM: HAEMORRHOIDS

The anus is lined with spongy tissue supplied with blood vessels – the anal cushions that enable the anus to close. This canal is a short, muscular tube with blood vessels that connects the rectum to the anus. Haemorrhoids, or in common terminology 'piles', are abnormal swellings of the vascular mucosa anal cushions around the anus. Essentially, they are swollen blood vessels. Internal piles start inside a person's anal canal which may at times protrude down out of the anus. Piles usually look like small, round, discoloured lumps. External haemorrhoids originate further down the anal canal, closer to the anus – they can be painful, especially if they have a blood clot in them, and accompanied by itchiness.

The incidence is unclear. Some dated community-based studies in the UK reported that haemorrhoids affect 13–36% of the general population (Lohsiriwat, 2012). Furthermore, in a recent systematic review van Tol et al. (2020) reported white people and people of higher socioeconomic status were affected more frequently than black people and people of lower socioeconomic status, possibly reflecting differences in health-seeking behaviour rather than a variation in prevalence. Women are predisposed to developing haemorrhoids during pregnancy though it's not clear what causes them. Triggers to increase likelihood of developing piles include:

- Constipation
- Straining when emptying the bowels
- Heavy lifting
- Pregnancy

Piles don't always cause pain or other symptoms and vary hugely between individuals, however some symptoms reported include:

- Bleeding when defecating (frank red blood) on toilet paper or on the surface of the faeces
- A lump in or around the anus
- A mucus discharge from the anus
- A feeling of anal 'fullness' and discomfort or a feeling of incomplete defecation or emptying of the bowels
- Itch or soreness on the anal area
- Pain and discomfort following defecation

Alongside treatments any presumed risks are recommended to be addressed, i.e. avoiding straining (with stool softeners), avoiding constipation (see section on constipation later in the chapter) or simple analgesia if pain is experienced. Piles may also be caused by problems such as inflammatory bowel disease, anal cancer, bowel cancer and anal fissures which ought to be excluded prior to the topical treatments suggested by the BNF or the pharmacists outlined in the following monographs.

Drug group: Topical steroid

Drug name: Benzyl benzoate with bismuth oxide, bismuth subgallate, hydrocortisone acetate, peru balsam and zinc oxide

UK brand names: Anusol

Average doses:

- Suppository – one suppository into the anus at night, in the morning and after each evacuation up to a maximum of three per day for a maximum period of one week; cream – apply sparingly in anal region each morning and after bowel movements; ointment (same as cream – may have a nozzle for anal insertion of cream/ointment)

What form does it come in: Cream, suppository, ointment

Duration of therapy: Symptomatic use – maximum of one week

Does it interact with other medicines: None reported however caution is recommended with other steroids used concurrently.

Drug group: Local anaesthetic and steroid

Drug name: Cinchocaine with hydrocortisone

UK brand names: Proctosedyl

Average doses:

- Ointment: Apply sparingly (thin layer) twice daily morning and night and after a bowel movement. Apply externally or by rectum. Suppository - one inserted into the anus night and morning and after a bowel movement.

What form does it come in: Suppository, ointment

Duration of therapy: Symptomatic. No longer than 7 days

Does it interact with other medicines: None reported however caution is recommended with other steroids used concurrently.

Drug name: Hydrocortisone (5%) with lidocaine (0.275%)

UK brand names: Xyloproct

Average doses:

- Spray - 1 spray up to three times a day to anal area; ointment - thin layer (sparingly) three times a day to anal area

What form does it come in: Spray, ointment

Duration of therapy: No more than 7 days

Does it interact with other medicines: None reported however caution is recommended with other steroids used concurrently. Steroids can cross the rectum and enter the systemic circulation.

Drug group: Opioid

Drug name: Kaolin (1 g) with morphine (0.458 mg per 5 ml dose)

UK brand names: None

(Continued)

Average doses:

- 10 ml every 6 hours, dose to be given in water

What form does it come in: Oral suspension

Duration of therapy: As short a duration as possible

Does it interact with other medicines: Yes, the interactions for morphine are the same as outlined in Chapter 7. The interactions for kaolin are:

- Decreased absorption of certain antimicrobial agents:
  o Chloroquine
  o Doxycycline
  o Eravacycline
  o Hydroxychloroquine
  o Lymecycline
  o Minaycline
  o Oxytetracycline
  o Tertracycline.

Caution: Kaolin is contraindicated in intestinal obstruction. The product contains a very small amount of morphine and thus theoretically it should be contraindicated in the same conditions as other morphine-containing preparations.

SYMPTOM: INDIGESTION AND HEARTBURN: DYSPEPSIA

There are a number of reasons why patients need to take indigestion medicines.

- Occasional, mild bouts of indigestion. Most people experience this once in a while often triggered by type of food (spicy) or certain factors such as being overweight or stressed which can make it worse.
- Indigestion during pregnancy. This is common and certain over-the-counter indigestion medicines are ok to take during pregnancy (with the guidance of the midwife or pharmacist).
- Long-term digestive problems. These may be pathologies such as: gastro-oesophageal reflux disease or peptic ulcers and may require stronger prescribed indigestion medicines.

Drugs that may also cause dyspepsia, such as alpha blockers, antimuscarinics, aspirin, benzodiazepines, beta blockers. Following investigation and exploration for an underlying condition, treatment may be one the three main types of medicine for indigestion or other approaches (i.e. lifestyle – smoking cessation etc.). The medicine groups are:

- Antacids and alginates
- Proton pump inhibitors
- H2 blockers famotidine and ranitidine

Drug group: Antacids and alginates

Drug name: Calcium carbonate

UK brand names: Settlers, Rennie, Calcichew

Average doses:

- 500 mg (1 tablet)

What form does it come in: Tablet, chewable tablet, effervescent tablet

Does it interact with other medicines: Yes, the following interactions are known:

- Chloroquine (oral) accentuated levels.
- Ciprofloxacin – decreased absorption with concurrent use.
- Eltrombopag – absorption impaired.
- Estramustine (anti-cancer) absorption impaired.
- Raltegravir (HIV medicine) decreased absorption.
- Medicines which increase serum calcium may result in hypercalcaemia (theoretical).

Caution: In people with high calcium or kidney stones (nephrolithiasis) due to effect of additional calcium and exacerbating the condition.

Drug name: Sodium alginate with potassium bicarbonate

UK brand names: Gaviscon, Acidex

Average doses:

- 1–2 tablets, to be chewed after meals and at bedtime, maximum four times a day. (Each tablet: sodium alginate 250 mg, sodium bicarbonate 106.5 mg and calcium carbonate 187.5 mg)

What form does it come in: Chewable tablet, oral suspension

Does it interact with other medicines: Yes, the following interactions are known:

- Chloroquine (oral) accentuated levels.
- Ciprofloxacin – decreased absorption with concurrent use.
- Eltrombopag – absorption impaired.
- Estramustine (anti-cancer) absorption impaired.
- Raltegravir (HIV medicine) decreased absorption.
- Medicines which increase serum calcium may result in hypercalcaemia (theoretical).

Caution: Some medicines need a 2-hour delay before taking if taken after antacids.

(Continued)

Drug name: Co-magaldrox

UK brand names: Maalox, Mucogel

Average doses:

- 10-20 ml, to be taken 20-60 minutes after meals, and at bedtime or when required

What form does it come in: Suspension

Does it interact with other medicines: Yes, the following interactions are known:

- Amlodipine - potentiates hypotension.
- Chloroquine - absorption decreased.
- Nitrofurantoin - absorption decreased.
- Risedronate - absorption decreased.

Caution: Antacids are known to interfere with the absorption of drugs such as tetracyclines, vitamins, ciprofloxacin, ketoconazole, levothyroxine, hydroxychloroquine, chloroquine, chlorpromazine, rifampicin, cefdinir, cefpodoxime, rosuvastatin.

Drug group: Proton pump inhibitors

Drug name: Omeprazole

UK brand names: Losec, Mezzopram

Average doses:

- 20 mg once a day (severe symptoms 40 mg once a day)

What form does it come in: Gastro-resistant tablet, gastro-resistant capsule, oral suspension, powder for solution for infusion

Does it interact with other medicines: Yes, the following interactions are known:

- Atazanavir, rilpivirine, tipranivir (HIV medicine) - reduces absorption.
- Bosutinib, dasatinib, (cancer medicine) - reduces absorption.
- Cenobamate (seizures) - enhances omeprazole.
- Citalopram (depression) - enhances effects.
- Clopidogrel (anti-thrombotic) - decrease effect.

- Escitalopram (depression) – enhances effect.
- Itraconazole and ketoconazle – (antifungal) – impaired absorption.
- Methotrexate (cancer) decreases elimination so enhances effects.

Caution: May impair absorption of acidic drugs due to being alkali.

Drug name: Esomeprazole

UK brand names: Nexium

Average doses:

- 20 mg once daily

What form does it come in: Gastro-resistant tablet, gastro-resistant capsule, gastro-resistant granules, powder for solution for injection

Does it interact with other medicines: Yes, the following interactions are known:

- as for omeprazole

Caution: As for omeprazole.

Drug group: H2 blockers

Drug name: Famotidine

UK brand names: None

Average doses:

- 20 mg once daily, dose to be taken at night

What form does it come in: Tablets

Does it interact with other medicines: Yes, as for omeprazole

Caution: H2 receptor antagonists might mask symptoms of gastric cancer; during pregnancy and breastfeeding – passes into breast milk so not advised.

(Continued)

Drug name: Ranitidine

UK brand names: Ranicalm

Average doses:

- 150 mg twice daily for 4-8 weeks, alternatively 300 mg once daily for 4-8 weeks, dose to be taken at night.

What form does it come in: Tablet, oral solution

Does it interact with other medicines: Yes, as for omeprazole.

Caution: H2 receptor antagonists might mask symptoms of gastric cancer.

Drug name: Cimetidine

UK brand names: Tagamet

Average doses:

- 400 mg twice daily for at least four weeks, to be taken with breakfast and at night

What form does it come in: Tablet, oral solution

Does it interact with other medicines: Yes, as for omeprazole.

Caution: As for ranitidine.

SYMPTOM: INFREQUENT MIGRAINE

Headaches such as migraine are a frequent cause of people seeking support and medical treatment. As a condition dominated by pain it is therefore a uniquely individual experience. There are many different types of headache (or head pain), some of these are classified in the pattern of presenting or in the causes or triggers attributed to them. Some of the most common types include:

Tension headaches: where pain spreads across both sides of the head, often starting at the back then progressing to the front. This is the most common form of headache pain and is often believed to be caused by eyestrain, stress or hunger. These can be acute or chronic and treated with simple analgesia (see Chapter 7).

Sinus headaches: this type of head pain results from nasal congestion and swelling in the sinus passages often felt behind the cheeks, nose and eyes. The pain worsens on bending forward, coughing or on first waking in the morning.

Cluster headaches: this is where the head pain occurs in 'clusters', a pattern such as being triggered daily by physical exertion, bright lights or even altitude. It may be due to dilation of the blood vessels of the brain due to a release of serotonin and histamines.

Medication-overuse headache: this is head pain due to the persistent regular use of simple analgesia (paracetamol) dosing for more than 15 days per month which can result in a 'rebound' effect. This is outlined further in Chapter 7.

There are several others – exercise headaches, pregnancy headaches etc. – pointing to a vast range in the population.

Migraine is the third most common health condition in the world. It is usually described as an intense pounding headache that can last for hours or even days. It is also referred to as a periodic, usually unilateral, throbbing form of headache often accompanied by nausea and vomiting. Migraine headaches can affect all age groups and their prevalence is difficult to establish, but estimates indicate around 10 million adults in the UK are affected (between 15% and 23% of the adult population; The Migraine Trust, 2020). The International Classification of Headache Disorders, recognised by the World Health Organization (WHO, 2016), identifies several types of migraine. The most common types are migraine with aura, migraine without aura and migraine aura without headache. The term 'aura' usually refers to sensory or visual disturbances including coloured spots, blind spots and flashing lights in front of the eyes.

Migraine may have an inherited tendency, and the headaches may be accompanied with sensory disturbance (aura). It is postulated that it is an instability in the way the brain deals with incoming sensory information, and that instability can become influenced by physiological changes like sleep, exercise and hunger (The Migraine Trust, 2020). There is currently no cure for migraines, although a number of treatments are available to help ease the symptoms. Triggers if known are suggested to be avoided, e.g. alcohol and stress, if possible. The key aims of medication are to stop the migraine attack, or to significantly reduce the severity of the headache and other associated symptoms, or be preventative, reducing the frequency, severity and duration of migraine attacks, and the development of medication-overuse headache. The key medicines in use here include:

- Monotherapy: a simple analgesic such as aspirin, paracetamol, ibuprofen (see Chapter 7) or a 5HT1-receptor agonist (also called a 'triptan').
  - Sumatriptan is the 5HT1-receptor agonist of choice.
  - Alternative 5HT1-receptor agonists include almotriptan, eletriptan, frovatriptan, naratriptan, rizatriptan and zolmitriptan.
- Non-steroidal anti inflammatories (NSAIDs): tolfenamic acid, diclofenac potassium, Mefenamic acid (menstrual migraine). See Chapter 7 for these medicines.
- Antiemetics, metoclopramide hydrochloride or prochlorperazine (see section below on nausea and vomiting).
- Preventative: Beta blockers, e.g. Propranolol hydrochloride, metoprolol tartrate (see Chapter 6). Topiramate is also used for migraine preventions but has other licensed uses (for seizures) too.

Drug group: Triptans

Drug name: Sumatriptan

UK brand names: Imigran

Average doses:

- Oral: initially 50-100 mg for 1 dose, followed by 50-100 mg after at least 2 hours if required, to be taken only if migraine recurs (patient not responding to initial dose should not take second dose for same attack); maximum 300 mg per day
- Intranasal spray: initially 10-20 mg, to be administered into one nostril, followed by 10-20 mg after at least 2 hours if required, to be taken only if migraine recurs (patient not responding to initial dose should not take second dose for same attack); maximum 40 mg per day
- Subcutaneous injection: initially 3-6 mg for 1 dose, followed by 3-6 mg after at least 1 hour if required, to be taken only if migraine recurs (patient not responding to initial dose should not take second dose for same attack), dose to be administered using an auto-injector; maximum 12 mg per day

What form does it come in: Tablet, solution for injections, spray

Does it interact with other medicines: Yes, the following serious interactions are known:

- Serotonin syndrome is a risk if used with antidepressants or antiemetics which alter serotonin level (5-HT); specific examples include:
  o Bupropion
  o Citalopram
  o Clomipramine
  o Dapoxitine
  o Dexamfetamine
  o Ergotamine
  o Escitalopram
  o Fentanyl
  o Granisetron
  o Tapentadol
  o Tramadol
  o Tryptofan
  o Phenelzine - increases level of sumatriptan.

Drug name: Topiramate

UK brand names: Topamax

Average doses:

- Initially 25 mg once daily for one week, dose to be taken at night, then increased in steps of 25 mg every week; usual dose 50–100 mg daily in 2 divided doses; maximum 200 mg per day

What form does it come in: Tablet, capsule, oral suspension

Does it interact with other medicines: Yes, the following serious interactions are known:

- Decreased efficacy of the following:
  - Hormones:
    - Combined hormonal contraceptives
    - Cyproterone
    - Desogestrel
    - Estrodial
    - Etonogestrel
    - Hormone replacement therapy
    - Levonorgestrel
    - Norethisterone
    - Ulipristal (emergency contraceptive)
  - Iminitib (for cancer).
- Enhanced effect if taken with:
  - Fosphenytoin (anti-seizure)
  - Valproate
  - Zonisamide.

Drug name: Sodium valproate

UK brand names: Epilim

Average doses:

- Oral (immediate release preparation). Initially 200 mg twice daily, then increased if necessary to 1.2–1.5 g daily in divided doses

What form does it come in: Tablet, modified-release tablet, gastro-resistant tablet, modified-release capsule, modified-release granules, oral solution, solution for injection, powder and solvent for solution for injection

(Continued)

Does it interact with other medicines: Yes, more than 70 interactions are reported. The following serious interactions are known:

- Acetazolamide (for high intraocular pressure) increased risk of valproate toxicity.
- Bupropion, nortriptyline (antidepressant): increased exposure when used with valproate.
- Ertapenem, imipenem (beta-lactam antibiotic): decreases the concentration of valproate.
- Fosphenytoin, phenytoin, primidone (anticonvulsive): decreases the concentration of valproate.
- Lamotrigine, topiramate (anticonvulsive): increased exposure in presence of valproate.
- Nirmatrelvir, ritonavir (antiviral): decrease the concentration of valproate.
- Olanzapine (antipsychotic): increased risk of adverse effects in presence of valproate.
- Propofol (anaesthesia): concentration increased with valproate.

Caution: Use in pregnancy and breastfeeding as it crosses the placental barrier or is present in breast milk.

SYMPTOM: MILD OR INFREQUENT CONSTIPATION

The incidence of mild or infrequent constipation is unknown. Chronic constipation however is highly prevalent, affecting between 10% and 15% of the population (Aziz et al., 2020). People with problematic constipation are explored for causative or pathological causes such as: irritable bowel or physiological dysfunction or drug (e.g. opioid) induced constipation. The initial management approach for these disorders is similar, focusing on diet, lifestyle and the use of standard over-the-counter laxatives. Treatments for constipations with laxatives are useful yet patients also need to be mindful that any persistent symptoms do need further attention, especially since drugs like laxatives do not suit everyone and may not aid in normalising bowel routines or actions. They are useful for short periods alongside lifestyle changes or if worsening encouraged to seek further medical support and advice.

Medicines used to treat mild constipation can be purchased in pharmacies over the counter or may be administered to patients in the community or other clinical areas.

There are four types of laxatives:

- **Bulk-forming laxatives** which work by increasing the mass or bulk of faeces within the bowel which can aid in stimulation to defecate (pass faeces).
- **Osmotic laxatives** which work by holding and diverting water from being absorbed and contributing to the bulk of the faeces enabling it to soften and pass more easily.
- **Stimulant laxatives** which work by stimulating the nerves within the colon to contract and thus expel the faeces out.
- **Stool softeners** which work by adding to the fluid content of hard, dry faeces (stools), making them easier to pass.

Stimulant laxatives will work quicker than the other types and the choice is up to the individual and in consultation with the pharmacist. If patients rely on laxatives or overuse them then problems can occur such as diarrhoea or impairment of absorption of other drugs, hence it is important for nurses to also know when and how to guide patients using laxatives.

Drug group: Bulk-forming laxative

Drug name: Ispaghula husk

UK brand names: Fybogel, YourFIBRE High-Fibre

Average doses:

- 1 sachet (3.5g isphagula husk) in 150 ml water. Once or twice daily as long as symptoms persist. Recommended to be given dissolved in water preferably taken after food and not within 90 minutes of other medicines

What form does it come in: Granules, effervescent granules

Does it interact with other medicines: No

Caution: Duration of therapy is as long as required or unless hypersensitivity or side effects occur (e.g. abdominal bloating/distention).

Drug group: Antispasmodic and bulk-forming laxative

Drug name: Fybogel Mebeverine

UK brand names: None

Average doses:

- 1 sachet (3.5g and 135 mg mebeverine hydrochloride) in 150 ml water. Once or twice daily as long as symptoms persist. Recommended to be given dissolved in water preferably taken after food and not within 90 minutes of other medicines

What form does it come in: Granules, effervescent granules

Does it interact with other medicines: No

Drug group: Osmotic laxative

Drug name: Lactulose

UK brand names: Duphalac

Average doses:

- 30-45 ml (starting dose) then 15 ml twice daily (maintenance dose) once or twice daily as long as symptoms persist

What form does it come in: Oral suspension, sachet powder (to dissolve)

Does it interact with other medicines: Yes, the following interactions are known:

- May increase the loss of potassium induced by other drugs (e.g. thiazides, steroids and amphotericin B).

Drug group: Stimulant laxative

Drug name: Bisacodyl

UK brand names: Dulcolax

Average doses: Oral: 5-10 mg once daily, dose to be taken at night; increased if necessary up to 20 mg once daily, dose to be taken at night. Rectally: 10 mg once daily, dose to be taken in the morning.

What form does it come in: Tablets, suppositories

Does it interact with other medicines: No

Cautions: Concerns over overuse or misuse means there are pack size restriction when purchasing OTC. IT is recommended dietary and lifestyle measures should be used first-line for relieving short-term occasional constipation, and that stimulant laxatives should only be used if these measures and other laxatives (bulk-forming and osmotic) are ineffective.

Drug name: Senna

UK brand names: Senakot, Senease,

Average doses: 7.5-15 mg once daily, dose usually taken at bedtime, initial dose should be low then gradually increased, higher doses up to 30 mg once daily may be prescribed under medical supervision.

What form does it come in: Tablets, oral solution

Does it interact with other medicines: No

Cautions: same as for biscodyl

Drug name: Co-danthrusate

UK brand names: none

Average doses: 5-15 mL once daily, to be taken at night.

What form does it come in: oral suspension

Does it interact with other medicines: Yes

- Baloxavir marboxil (antiviral – influenza) increased by dicusate. Theoretical interaction.

Cautions: Avoid in patients with intestinal obstructions.

Drug name: Sodium picosulfate

UK brand names: Dulcolax pico

Average doses: 5-10 mg once daily, dose to be taken at bedtime.

What form does it come in: oral suspension

Does it interact with other medicines: Yes

- Baloxavir marboxil (antiviral – influenza) may be increased. Theoretical interaction.

Cautions: Avoid in patients with intestinal obstructions.

Drug group: Stool softener

Drug name: Docusate sodium

UK brand names: Dioctyl

Average doses: Oral: 100 mg 3 times a day, dose can be increased if necessary up to maximum 500 mg daily in divided doses (until chronic constipation eases). Rectally: 120 mg for 1 dose.

(Continued)

What form does it come in: Tablets, suppositories

Does it interact with other medicines: Yes

- Baloxavir marboxil (antiviral – influenza) increased by docusate. Theoretical interaction.

Cautions: Avoid in patients with intestinal obstructions.

Drug name: Glycerol

UK brand names: Glycerin

Average doses: 4g as required

What form does it come in: suppositories

Does it interact with other medicines: No

SYMPTOM: NAUSEA AND VOMITING

Nausea is considered to act as a protective mechanism, a warning to avoid ingesting potential toxins. However, it is a common symptom at times associated with other interventions or behaviours such as post-operatively, chemotherapy-induced nausea and motion sickness. It is often thought to be a precursor to the act of vomiting and whilst it might be in some situations, for example in gastroenteritis (stomach influenza), there is no explicit or direct relationship. One could argue nausea is subjective and vomiting (or expelling enteral products through the mouth) is mechanical. Most people with nausea describe it as more disabling, feeling worse and lasting longer than vomiting. Stimuli causing nausea and vomiting originate from organs (visceral), inner ear (vestibular) and central nervous system locations (chemoreceptor trigger zone or CTZ). These alter balances of nerve chemicals such as serotonin/dopamine, histamine/acetylcholine and serotonin/dopamine, resulting in the subjective response, nausea. This explains the current pharmacological approach for nausea and vomiting. Antiemetics however are generally only prescribed when the cause of vomiting is known as indicated in the BNF (JFC, 2023), such as after cancer chemotherapy or post-operatively. The key groups of medicines used in this category are antihistamines, phenothiazines, serotonin (5HT3-receptor) antagonists and medicines which act on the central CTZ.

- Antihistamines, e.g. cinnarizine, cyclizine, (promethazine hydrochloride; see Chapter 2).
- Phenothiazines, e.g. chlorpromazine hydrochloride, prochlorperazine, trifluoperazine.
- Metoclopramide hydrochloride.
- 5HT3-receptor antagonists, e.g. granisetron, ondansetron and palonosetron.

Drug group: Antihistamines

Drug name: Cinnarizine

UK brand names: Stugeron

Average doses:

- 30 mg three times a day. For motion or travel sickness: initially 30 mg, dose to be taken 2 hours before travel, then 15 mg every 8 hours if required, dose to be taken during journey

What form does it come in: Tablet

Does it interact with other medicines: Yes, the BNF reports 122 interactions. The following serious interactions are known:

- Antidepressant group: if combined has depressant effects: amitriptyline; chlorpromazine; doxepin.
- Opioids: alfentanil: depressant effects and impaired skills (e.g. driving).
- Isocarboxazid, phenelzine (antidepressant): risk of antimuscarinic effects, e.g. constipation, transient bradycardia, arrhythmias, reduced bronchial secretions, urinary retention, dilation of the pupils, dry mouth, flushing, and dryness of the skin.
- Benzodiaepines: midazelam, mirtazapine, alprazolam: depressant effects and impaired skills (e.g. driving).
- Baclofen (antispasmodic) depressant effects and impaired skills (e.g. driving).
- Alcohol: depressant effects and impaired skills (e.g. driving).

Drug name: Cyclizine

UK brand names: Cyclizine

Average doses:

- 50 mg three times a day

What form does it come in: Tablet, solution for injection

Does it interact with other medicines: Yes, the BNF reports 152 interactions. The following serious interactions are known:

- As for cinnarizine.
- Clozapine (anti schizophrenic) - risk of intestinal obstruction.

Drug group: Phenothiazines

Drug name: Prochlorperazine

UK brand names: Stemetil

Average doses:

- 12.5 mg as required (nausea and vomiting); 5-15 mg daily (labyrinthine disorders) decreased when resolved

What form does it come in: Tablet, buccal tablet, oral solution, solution for injection

Does it interact with other medicines: Yes, more than 250 interactions are noted in the BNF. The following serious interactions are indicated:

- Alcohol - causes hypotension.
- Alprazolam. - cause sedation
- Amitriptyline - risk of hypotension.
- Clozapine (antipsychotic) - anti-muscarinic effects: constipation and risk of intestinal obstruction; tachycardia, nervous system depressant.
- Levodopa (Parkinson's disease) - decreased effect.
- Lithium - neurotoxicity.
- Phenelzine, tranylcypromine (mental health medicines) - severe hypotension risk.

Caution: This drug is also prescribed as an antipsychotic medicine for agitation, aggression and distress so caution is needed with other antipsychotic medicines. Pregnancy and breastfeeding: If prescribing prochlorperazine in the third trimester the neonate ought to be monitored for side effects such as agitation, hypertonia, hypotonia, tremor, drowsiness, feeding problems and respiratory distress.

Drug name: Chlorpromazine hydrochloride

UK brand names: None

Average doses:

- 10-25 mg every 4-6 hours (mostly in palliative care)

What form does it come in: Tablet, oral solution and suppository

Does it interact with other medicines: Yes, more than 250 interactions are noted in the BNF. See prochlorperazine.

Caution: This drug is also prescribed as an antipsychotic medicine for agitation, aggression and distress so caution is needed with other antipsychotic medicines.

Drug name: Metoclopramide hydrochloride

UK brand names: Maxolon

Average doses:

- 10 mg up to three times a day

What form does it come in: Tablet, oral solution, solution for injection

Does it interact with other medicines: Yes, the following serious interactions are known:

- Levodopa (Parkinson's disease) - effects decreased.
- Mivacurium, prilocaine (anaesthesia) - risk of methaemoglobinaemia (blood).
- Posaconazole (antifungal) - absorption decreased.

Caution: Not licensed for use in migraine but occasionally is prescribed. Potentially inappropriate for elderly patients with Parkinson's disease due to alteration of dopamine levels.

Drug name: Domperidone

UK brand names: Motilium

Average doses:

- 10 mg up to three times a day for a maximum of one week

What form does it come in: Tablet, oral suspension

Does it interact with other medicines: Yes, the BNF states there are 98 interactions. The following serious interactions are known:

- The following interact with domperidone leading to cardiac arrythmia issues (prolonged QT intervals):
  - Disopyramide, hydroquinidine, quinidine (antiarrhythmics)
  - Amiodarone, dronedarone, ibutilide, sotalol (antiarrhythmics)
  - Haloperidol, pimozide, sertindole, chlorpromazine (antipsychotics)
  - Citalopram, escitalopram (antidepressants)
  - Erythromycin, levofloxacin, moxifloxacin, clarithromycin (antibiotics)
  - Pentamidine (antifungal agents)
  - Toremifene, vandetanib, apalutamide (cancer medicines)
  - Methadone (for opioid dependence, pain)
  - Ondansetron (anti-emetic in cancer)
  - Quinine (antimalarial).

(Continued)

- Bromocriptine (for prolactin lowering) – effect decreased.
- Fosamprenavir (HIV medicine) – increases levels of domperidone.
- Itraconazole, ketoconazole (antifungal) – increases levels of domperidone.

Drug name: Granisetron

UK brand names: Kytril

Average doses:

Cancer treatment:

- Orally 1–2 mg, taken within 1 hour before treatment, then 2 mg daily in 1–2 divided doses for up to a week following treatment
- Transdermal patch – 3.1 mg patch (24 hour duration) on upper arm 24–48 hours before treatment and 24 hours after treatment
- Intravenous – 10–40 micrograms/kg (maximum per dose 3 mg), to be given 5 minutes before start of treatment, then as required to a maximum of 9 mg per day

Post-operative nausea: Intravenous – 1 mg, diluted to 5 ml and given over 30 seconds; maximum 3 mg per day.

What form does it come in: Tablet, solution for injection, transdermal patch

Does it interact with other medicines: Yes, the BNF indicates 115 interactions. The following serious interactions are known:

- Same as for domperidone in relation to cardiac arrythmia issues (prolonged QT intervals).

GO FURTHER

It has been indicated that some drugs have a link with a neurotransmitter called acetylcholine that is they may act as blockers of this chemical and are termed antimuscarinics. This article reviews acetylcholine and its functions to better understand the 'antimuscarinic effects' mentioned: Aliouche, H. (2020) What is acetylcholine? Available at: www.news-medical.net/health/What-is-Acetylcholine.aspx

MEDICINES IN PREGNANCY AND BREASTFEEDING

The range of commonly available medicines found within this chapter indicates a huge potential for problems during pregnancy or when breastfeeding. Over-the-counter medications still contain active ingredients which may cross the placenta or pass through to breast milk. The common symptoms associated with pregnancy such as dyspepsia or constipation or aches and pains may be relieved with medicines, but this ought to be approached with caution. Some medicines which are topical carry less risk and may be advised as suitable for pregnancy as they act only on the local area, for example topical haemorrhoidal preparations. These are licensed for use during pregnancy or breastfeeding as they do not enter the systemic circulation. Other medicines require further cautions or have limited safety information and are best avoided. Conditions such as migraine may worsen in pregnancy and there is limited evidence of the effect of using 5HT1-receptor agonists during pregnancy. There is a reported increased risk of major congenital malformations, (MHRA, 2022) and intra-uterine growth restriction has been seen with topiramate, and as such the advice is that they should be avoided unless the potential benefit outweighs the risk. In a breastfeeding situation the guidance is to pace this with feeding, e.g. avoid breastfeeding for a period of time after taking the medications as it crosses in milk.

The use of sedating antihistamines in the latter part of the third trimester may cause adverse effects in neonates such as irritability, paradoxical excitability and tremor. Most anti-histamines are present in breast milk in varying amounts; although not known to be harmful, most manufacturers advise avoiding their use while breastfeeding.

LEARNING FROM A CASE STUDY: TEST YOUR KNOWLEDGE

Giovanni Argyll is 84 years old and has been brought to your practice by his wife to ask for advice on his recent constipation. On discussion with him it emerges he has recently been experiencing back pain, which prevents him from getting out and doing his usual activities. The GP gave him co-dydramol ten days ago and things are starting to improve, but he is still careful walking especially to the toilet at night. His wife says that she bought some little brown tablets in a pharmacy when she was constipated, but they gave her stomach pains. She tried to get him to take them, but he refuses. He thinks he should perhaps have something gentle like prunes, but they give him 'heartburn' and he already takes omeprazole for that.

1   Why do you think Mr Argyll may have had constipation recently?
2   What sort of laxative do you think Mrs Argyll has been taking? Is this the most appropriate? Explain your answer.
3   What guidance could you give Mr Argyll on managing his symptoms?

IF I REMEMBER 5 THINGS FROM THIS CHAPTER:

1   'Common symptoms' refers to a wide range of expressions of symptoms which may be simple, short lived or occur due to life stresses, vulnerabilities or behavioural choices, e.g. vulnerability to pollen (hayfever) or travel sickness.

2   Medicines to alleviate such common symptoms are available either on prescription or without prescription OTC at pharmacies.

3   Signs and symptoms are features aligned with disease and disorder processes and may be unique to a disease or disorder (e.g. growths) or broader than that.

4   Medicines all have active ingredients and potential interactions which can be an issue with self-purchased and self-administered (i.e. OTC) alongside prescribed or other medications.

5   There are more than 35 common symptoms or minor or self-limiting conditions which can be treated with self-administered mediations ranging from allergies to motion sickness to fungal infections.

ANSWERS TO CASE STUDY QUESTIONS

1   a) Mr Argyll is elderly, however age is not a cause of constipation; his lifestyle factors such as decreased mobility, decreased fluid intake (i.e. walking to the toilet at night) and potentially decreased dietary intake may promote constipation in this case. b) Mr Argyll has recently had back pain, which may have further decreased his mobility. c) Mr Argyll has been taking dihydrocodeine (as part of co-dydramol), one of the adverse effects of which is constipation.

2   From the description of the adverse effects, this seems most likely to be 'senna' a stimulating laxative, as this is associated with abdominal cramps as an effect. If so, yes this is appropriate for Mr Argyll. Stimulant laxatives have the advantage of being fairly quick acting to counteract the decreased bowel motility effects of the opioid analgesics. They are also useful for occasional use. There are other laxatives which may be used:

   o   Bulk-forming laxatives (such as ispaghula husk), useful in a diet lacking in fibre (but not to replace dietary fibre).

   o   Faecal softeners (such as docusate).

   o   Osmotic laxatives (such as lactulose); however, it is essential that fluid intake is maintained during their use.

3   a) Lifestyle measures such as increased dietary fibre, fluid intake, keeping as mobile as possible, etc. b) A laxative would seem appropriate at this stage as it is likely that his constipation is drug-induced. Discuss the benefits of senna, and he could try starting with one tablet to minimise the adverse effects. If he is reluctant to try senna he could be encouraged to use lactulose but it may take 48 hours to work. c) His omeprazole may also cause constipation, so he ought to discuss this with his GP. d) Ensure he understands

his co-dydramol has side effects and whilst it may be short term, he could discuss the constipation with his GP and a possible alternative analgesic.

REFERENCES AND RECOMMENDED READING

Aziz, I., Whitehead, W.E., Palsson, O.S., Törnblom, H. and Simrén, M. (2020) An approach to the diagnosis and management of Rome IV functional disorders of chronic constipation. *Expert Review Gastroenterology and Hepatology*, *14*(1): 39–46. doi:10.1080/ 17474124.2020.1708718

Barrett, B. (2018) Viral Upper Respiratory Infection. *Integrative Medicine*, 170–179.e7. doi: 10.1016/B978-0-323-35868-2.00018-9.

British Medical Association (BMA) (2019) Over-the-counter medicines guidance. General Practitioners Committee. Available at: www.bma.org.uk/media/1548/bma-otc-medicine-guidance-march-2019.pdf

International Headache Society (2018) International classification of headache disorders (ICHD-3). *Cephalalgia*, *38*(1): 1–211. https://ichd-3.org/wp-content/uploads/2018/01/The-International-Classification-of-Headache-Disorders-3rd-Edition-2018.pdf

Joint Formulary Committee (JFC) (2023) *British National Formulary*. London: BMJ and Pharmaceutical Press. https://bnf.nice.org.uk/

Kenealy, T. (2014) Sore throat. Clinical evidence. Available at: www.ncbi.nlm.nih.gov/pmc/articles/PMC3948435/

Lohsiriwat, V. (2012) Hemorrhoids: From basic pathophysiology to clinical management. *World Journal of Gastroenterology*, *18*(17), 2009–2017.

Medicines and Healthcare Regulatory Authority (MHRA) (2022). Safety review to begin on topiramate. Available at: https://www.gov.uk/drug-safety-update/topiramate-topamax-start-of-safety-review-triggered-by-a-study-reporting-an-increased-risk-of-neurodevelopmental-disabilities-in-children-with-prenatal-exposure

National Institute for Health and Care Excellence (NICE) (2022) Clinical knowledge summaries: Sore throat – Acute. Available at: https://cks.nice.org.uk/topics/sore-throat-acute/

NHS England and Clinical Commissioners (2019) Items which should not routinely be prescribed in primary care: Guidance for CCGs. Available at: www.england.nhs.uk/wp-content/uploads/2019/08/items-which-should-not-routinely-be-prescribed-in-primary-care-v2.1.pdf

NHS England and Clinical Commissioners (2018) Conditions for which over the counter items should not routinely be prescribed in primary care: Guidance for CCGs. Available at: www.england.nhs.uk/wp-content/uploads/2018/03/otc-guidance-for-ccgs.pdf

NHS Inform (n.d.) Cough. Available at: www.nhsinform.scot/illnesses-and-conditions/lungs-and-airways/cough

Public Health England (PHE) (2022) Official statistics: Surveillance of influenza and other seasonal respiratory viruses in winter 2021 to 2022. Available at: www.gov.uk/government/

statistics/annual-flu-reports/surveillance-of-influenza-and-other-seasonal-respiratory-viruses-in-winter-2021-to-2022

The Migraine Trust (2020) *The State of the Migraine Nation: Who Is Living with Migraine in the UK?* Rapid Research Review. London: Migraine Trust.

van Tol, R.R., Kleijnen, J., Watson, A.J.M., Jongen, J., Altomare, D.F., Qvist, N., Higuero, T., Muris, J.W.M. and Breukink, S.O. (2020) European Society of ColoProctology: Guideline for haemorrhoidal disease. *Colorectal Disease*, *22*(6): 650–662. doi:10.1111/codi.14975.

World Health Organisation (WHO) (2016) Headache disorder. Available at: www.who.int/news-room/fact-sheets/detail/headache-disorders

9 MEDICINE CONSIDERATIONS IN SPECIAL POPULATIONS

RACHAEL MAJOR
SHEILA CUNNINGHAM

AFTER READING THIS CHAPTER YOU WILL BE ABLE TO:

- Recognise what is meant by the term special populations.
- Consider the differences in pharmacokinetics and pharmacodynamics in special populations.
- Recognise the risks of drug administration in special populations.
- Apply knowledge of special populations to clinical decision making in medicines management.

OVERVIEW

Certain groups of people need special consideration when it comes to drug administration due to physiological differences which cause additional vulnerabilities. These special populations are at a higher risk of injury (or in some cases lack of response) from drugs and therefore further monitoring, different dosages or different prescriptions may be required. Clinical trials may also be limited in some of these groups due to caution because of increased risks as well as participant biases (Grimsrud et al., 2015). Commonly recognised special populations include women (pregnant and non-pregnant), children (not addressed in this book), the elderly, people with learning disabilities and those receiving palliative care. Factors such as ethnicity, hepatic and renal impairment and weight may also influence the effectiveness of drug therapy and potential adverse drug reaction (ADRs) and therefore they are also addressed in this chapter.

Women

Although making up a significant proportion of the population, women, both pregnant and non-pregnant, can be viewed as a special population. Women demonstrate differences in pharmacokinetics when compared to men and this can influence how they respond to medicines, despite dose-related changes not generally being recommended in any of the prescribing guidelines. Women report more ADRs and may not have the most effective dose of the drugs as they are underrepresented in drug trials. Women have slower gastric emptying and gut transit than men, although alcohol is absorbed faster and at relatively higher concentrations than men due to reduced concentrations of the enzyme alcohol dehydrogenase in the stomach. Women generally have a higher percentage of body fat and lower body water content than men. Lipophilic drugs such as benzodiazepines and opioids have a higher half-life, as they accumulate in the fat, increasing the risks of overdose with extended use. Metabolism can also show sex-related differences in women and men as enzyme expression has been shown to be different, with these enzymes working at different rates. Renal blood flow and glomerular filtration rate is also higher in men compared with women, increasing excretion (Chu, 2014).

GO FURTHER

Interestingly, women show slower clearance of paracetamol than men. However, difference is offset if the woman is taking a combined oestrogen-progesterone oral contraceptive.

See Allegaert et al. (2015) Paracetamol pharmacokinetics and metabolism in young women. https://doi.org/10.1186/s12871-015-0144-3

Women also have a higher risk of impaired driving after taking zolpidem (used for insomnia) the night before, with the United States Food and Drug Administration (2018) recommending that dosages be reduced for women, although this has not been followed through in the United Kingdom.

Pregnancy and breastfeeding

Drugs can have a harmful effect on the foetus at any stage of pregnancy and therefore it is important to consider this when prescribing and administering medicines to women of childbearing age and men trying to conceive a child. Teratogenesis (when drugs cause congenital abnormalities) is most likely to occur in the first trimester of pregnancy, whereas in the second or third trimester, drugs are more likely to have a harmful effect on growth and development. It must also be remembered that drugs given just before or during delivery may also have an effect on the infant once they are born. In most cases, the decision to take medications during pregnancy must consider the benefit to the mother compared to the risk to the foetus and minimum dosages should be given.

Breastfeeding is known to have many benefits for both the infant and mother, however in many cases there is little information on the effects of drugs taken by the breastfeeding mother on the infant due to lack of research. Advice is often given on whether the drug is found in breast milk, with manufacturers tending to advise avoiding if this is the case, however the amount of drug found in breast milk may well not have an effect on the infant (Joint Formulary Committee, 2024).

Pregnancy and breastfeeding is addressed in most of the chapters within the specific drug groups.

Elderly

The elderly require additional care and attention when it comes to prescribing and drug administration. Ageing increases the risk of developing multiple diseases and the effects of normal ageing on the body reduces drug metabolism and excretion (see also the section on renal and hepatic impairment). Physical changes due to aging and disease may mean that they find it difficult to take medication, for example they may not be able to open medication packaging or bottles, or they may not be able to swallow tablets. Taking tablets without sufficient liquid or whilst reclined can lead to oesophageal ulceration.

Polypharmacy is common in the elderly and can cause a burden to older people and family carers, particularly if this includes complex regimens. More than one in four people over the age of 85 take at least ten different medications per week (Age UK, 2017). Polypharmacy is associated with increased adverse drug events and interactions and lack of concordance, with up to 50% of medicines for long-term conditions not being taken as intended and as many as 20% of prescribed medications not being appropriate (Age UK, 2017). In some cases, ADRs, the inability to manage the large volume of medications or complex drug routines can lead to no medication being taken at all. Medicine optimisation (see Chapter 1) is particularly important for older people.

Non-pharmacological approaches may be as effective as medicines in some cases, such as increasing movement for reducing gravitational oedema or social prescribing improving mood, combatting loneliness and stress.

The nervous system of the elderly is more sensitive to commonly used drugs and other organs such as kidneys are more susceptible to the effects of drugs. Acute illness, especially leading to dehydration, can make this problem worse and therefore the following drugs should be used with caution or at a lower dose:

- Warfarin
- Digoxin
- Opioid analgesics
- Benzodiazepines
- Antipsychotics
- Antiparkinsonian drugs
- NSAIDs

GO FURTHER

The STOP/START criteria are evidence-based tools to review medications specifically designed for people 65 or older. They give a list of drugs that should be reviewed in the elderly, along with a rationale.

Further details can be found here: www.england.nhs.uk/wp-content/uploads/2017/03/toolkit-general-practice-frailty-1.pdf

People with learning disabilities

People with learning disabilities are more likely to have poorer health and a lower life expectancy than the general population, and diagnostic overshadowing is a known problem. They are also more likely to have complex drug regimens and polypharmacy and less likely to recognise and report side effects (Royal Pharmaceutical Society, 2016). Overmedication of people with learning disabilities, especially with antipsychotic medication, has led to the campaign 'Stopping over medication of people with a learning disability, autism, or both' (STOMP) (NHS England 2016).

Consideration needs to be given to giving clear information to the person with learning disabilities in a form that they can understand and to involve carers where appropriate. This needs to include whether there are any dietary restrictions associated with the medication and if recreational drugs or alcohol should be avoided. Some people with learning disabilities may also have dysphagia and alternative routes of administration may include feeding tubes or liquid formulations. Crushing tablets or opening capsules may alter the pharmacokinetics of the drug and should be avoided, and covert administration avoided where possible and only considered in line with the Capacity Act (2005).

Difference or difficulties with communication can also increase risks associated with medication management for people with learning disabilities. For example, they may not be able to effectively communicate that they are experiencing illness, side effects or pain and behavioural changes may be the only noticeable sign. It is therefore really important that a person-centred approach to medication management is taken, involving the person with learning disabilities, their carers and those who know them well.

GO FURTHER

Public Health England has developed guidance about making reasonable adjustments for people with learning disabilities, which although written for pharmacies will help support nurses to deliver care.

This is available at: www.gov.uk/government/publications/pharmacy-and-people-with-learning-disabilities/pharmacy-and-people-with-learning-disabilities-making-reasonable-adjustments-to-services

---

Hepatic and renal impairment

The liver is the main route for metabolism of most drugs, either to active forms or inactive forms as part of elimination. The liver has a large reserve but in severe liver disease this may not occur effectively, and this will result in either lack of effect of the drug, or more commonly an accumulation and an increase in adverse effects. Some drugs can also increase the pathophysiology associated with severe liver disease, such as impaired blood clotting, fluid overload and hepatic encephalopathy. Warfarin, NSAIDs, corticosteroids, sedative drugs and opioids are some of these drugs which should be used with caution. Drugs that are known to be hepatotoxic (including paracetamol) should also be used with caution as even low doses may cause further damage. Drugs that are highly protein bound such as phenytoin and prednisolone can become more toxic due to low blood albumen levels associated with severe liver disease.

The kidneys are the main route of excretion for most drugs and therefore renal impairment will reduce clearance and increase concentrations of these in the body. This could lead to increased effects of these drugs, increased side effects and potential harm. Some patients with renal impairment have been found to be more sensitive to some drugs, even if elimination is not reduced (see the BNF). Kidney function reduces with age with two-thirds of 70–80-year-olds having around half the kidney function of a young adult (Wood et al., 2018). Lower doses of drugs are often recommended in renal impairment although it should be noted that estimated glomerular filtration rate has been shown to underestimate the degree of renal impairment in the elderly and be inaccurate in body builders, amputees, those with muscle-wasting diseases and vegans. Nephrotoxic drugs should be avoided where possible in renal disease to preserve remaining kidney function.

Common drugs that should be avoided or used with caution in renal impairment due to increased risk of toxicity, hyperkalaemia or nephrotoxicity (Whittaker et al., 2018; Willacy, 2022):

- NSAIDs
- ACE inhibitors
- Lithium
- Potassium supplements
- Potassium sparing diuretics
- Digoxin
- Anticonvulsants (especially phenytoin)
- H2 receptor antagonists
- Antibiotics (especially aminoglycosides such as gentamycin)
- Contrast media containing iodine
- Phosphate containing bowel preparation products

Palliative care

The aim of palliative and end-of-life care is to improve the quality of life of patients and to relieve suffering and distress, and should use a multidisciplinary approach. Specialist palliative care teams and hospice care teams can support patients and families through this stage of life using holistic approaches to the assessment of needs, care and treatment. Drug therapy in this stage of life aims to manage symptoms such as pain, anorexia, nausea, excessive respiratory secretions, dyspnoea, constipation, restlessness and confusion, insomnia, convulsions, muscle spasm or fungating tumours. Standard medications may be used differently in palliative care or 'off license'; for example antipsychotic drugs such as levomepromazine or haloperidol used to treat nausea as well as restlessness, agitation and confusion or distress.

In principle, the minimum number of drugs should be given, to reduce the complexity of the regimen, potential side effects and drug interactions and also the effort required to take them, but symptom control needs to be as effective as possible. Drugs that are no longer required or will have no benefit should also be stopped. As the end of life approaches, patients may no longer be able to swallow oral medications and the route of administration may need to be altered. The use of syringe drivers may be beneficial in these cases. Many patients wish to stay at home at the end of their life and this may also affect the choice of medications.

Patients are often concerned about pain at this stage of life. Pain caused by bone metastases can be treated with radiotherapy, bisphosphonates (see Chapter 5) or radioactive isotopes of strontium. Ketamine may be used to manage uncontrolled terminal pain at levels that are approaching anaesthetic doses. Further information on drugs for pain management can be found in Chapter 7.

Corticosteroids (see Chapter 3) such as prednisolone or dexamethasone can be useful for anorexia and breathlessness and dysphagia if there is bronchospasm or an obstruction due to a tumour. Dexamethasone can also be used to reduce intracranial pressure. Morphine can also be used to relieve dyspnoea.

GO FURTHER

If you want to know more about medicine management for palliative care patients at home, please review this article by Latif et al. (2020), available at: https://pharmaceutical-journal.com/article/ld/caring-for-palliative-care-patients-at-home-medicines-management-principles-and-considerations

For further information on medicines used in palliative care, an extensive evidence-based guide can be found on the Palliative Care Guidelines Plus website, available at: https://book.pallcare.info

---

Ethnicity

Race and ethnicity have been shown to affect both pharmacokinetics and pharmacodynamics, although the reasons for this are complex.

Pharmacogenetics may play a role in differences. There is evidence that there are differences in race-related expression of some genes which code for proteins involved in the metabolism of drugs. For example glucose-6-phosphate dehydrogenase deficiency is more common in people with an African, Middle Eastern, East Asian or Mediterranean heritage, and this can lead to high risks of haemolysis with a number of drugs such as antimalarial drugs, high dose aspirin, NSAIDs, quinidine, sulphur drugs, dapsone, prilocaine and some antibiotics such as quinolones and nitrofurantoin. Cytochrome P450 2D6 is an important enzyme in the metabolism of many drugs including codeine to its active metabolite morphine and there are a number of different genetic variations in the genes that code for that enzyme which lead to poor or ultra metabolisers. Poor metabolisers will have a more analgesic affect from codeine, whereas ultra metabolisers will produce more morphine, which can potentially lead to overdose. Research has shown that there are a higher percentage of ultra metabolisers in East African populations (20–29%) compared to Europeans (2–3%), with poor metabolisers found more commonly in Asians (approximately 12%) than Europeans (approximately 2%) (Koopmans et al., 2021).

Diet can play a role in absorption of drugs, with low-fat vegetarian diets reducing the rate of absorption of certain drugs such as paracetamol, possibly due to reduced gastric emptying (Olafuyi et al., 2021). Garlic can inhibit certain cytochrome P450 enzymes and traditional herbal medicines such as teas can also cause drug interactions (Izzo, 2012). It is therefore important to ask patients what other supplements, traditional medicines or herbs they are taking.

Current NICE guidelines (2022a) advise caution with the use of ACE inhibitors and angiotensin II receptor blockers in patients with African or Caribbean origin as they may response less well to them, with calcium channel blockers to be prescribed instead as first line treatment. There are however a number of authors questioning that approach, suggesting that this might actually be a harmful generalisation and that a personalised approach is more beneficial to the patient (Hunter et al., 2022; Sinnott et al., 2020). The expansion of pharmacogenomics will facilitate this.

Weight/size

Both being obese and very small or thin can change the way patients react to medicines or the drug concentration that they receive. In general adult dosages are based on average sized people with the same dose prescribed for all adults. Particular care needs to be taken when administering drugs with a narrow therapeutic index such as aminoglycosides (such as gentamicin), ciclosporin, carbamazepine, digoxin, digitoxin, flecainide, lithium, phenytoin, phenobarbital, rifampicin, theophylline and warfarin to calculate the risk of toxicity or under-dosing the patient. Some drugs are prescribed based on total body weight up to a maximum dose. Cefepime, a cephalosporin antibiotic, gives different doses for adults weighing under and over 41 kg whereas edoxaban, a factor xa inhibitor (see Chapter 6) gives different dosages for under and over 61 kg (Joint Formulary Committee, 2024).

Extreme obesity (a BMI of 40 kg/m^2 or more) increases the amount of fat in the body, lean body mass, organ size, cardiac output and blood pressure. The volume over which the drugs are distributed is also increased, although how drugs are distributed will depend on whether they are fat or water soluble. For drugs that are hydrophilic such as aminoglycosides, acyclovir, glycopeptides and low-molecular weight heparins, the amount of body fat will not affect available concentration of the drug, and ideal body weight, not actual body weight, should be used for dose calculations when administering aminoglycosides such as gentamycin, and serum gentamycin levels monitored closely. For drugs that are lipophilic, such as phenytoin, propranolol, midazolam, diazepam, verapamil and trazadone, it may take longer to get to a steady state of the drugs, the half-life may be longer and the drug may persist in the body for longer, increasing the risk of interactions, even after the drug has been discontinued (Bruno et al., 2021).

Obesity increases the likelihood of conditions that affect drug metabolism and excretion such as hepatic and renal impairment. Excretion may increase initially as glomerular filtration rate initially increases with obesity due to increased renal blood flow and pressure, although this may eventually lead to renal damage and reduced excretion.

Some drugs can also cause weight gain, either directly or as a side effect, and this can be distressing for some patients. Insulins, pioglitazone and sulfonylureas used to treat diabetes increase the storage of excess glucose as fat. Glucocorticoids cause water retention, increased appetite and fat redistribution, especially with chronic use, and oral contraceptives also can cause weight gain. Antipsychotics, selective serotonin reuptake inhibitors and tricyclic anti-depressants can also cause weight gain.

While a healthy diet, psychological support and exercise are recommended for weight loss, there are drugs that can be given when these measures alone are not effective, particularly in patients with a weight-related comorbidity, although the only drug currently recommended by NICE (2022b) is orlistat. This drug reduces the absorption of dietary fat therefore reducing calorie intake. Common side effects of abdominal pain, diarrhoea, fatty stools and even faecal incontinence can be reduced by reducing fat consumption.

Drug name: Orlistat

UK brand names: Allu, Beacita, Orlos, Xenical

Average doses:

- 120 mg immediately before, during or up to an hour after each main meal

What form does it come in: Capsule

Does it interact with other medicines: Yes, the following interactions are known:

- May affect the absorption of concurrently administered drugs – take separately, especially drugs with a narrow therapeutic index, antiepileptics and antiretrovirals.

GO FURTHER

A review article and interesting evidence on: Hypertension in women: A South-Asian perspective, by Farrukh et al. (2022): www.frontiersin.org/articles/10.3389/fcvm.2022.880374/full

Reflect on what this article indicates about ethnic and gender differences in medicines.

LEARNING FROM A CASE STUDY: TEST YOUR KNOWLEDGE

Lalita is a 47-year-old and comes to your clinic for periodic review of her blood pressure. She was diagnosed two years ago with hypertension which is prevalent in her family and appears to be controlled with amlodipine 5 mg daily. Her father had hypertension too and died when he was 55 years of a stroke in her home country Bangladesh, so Lalita is understandably anxious. Lalita is determined to control her blood pressure and has been exercising and losing weight but is still a little overweight with a body mass index of 29 kg/m². Today her blood pressure reads 145/85 mmHg and she is noticeably anxious so you wait to record her blood pressure again. She also complains of frequently feeling tired, at times dizzy, and having headaches which come on shortly after eating breakfast. She controls her headaches with paracetamol but finds she is taking them daily so wants a prescription for them. Her 15-year-old son is also being difficult and playing truant from school. To top it all she thinks she is menopausal and with the worry has missed her last two menstrual periods; if only her daily glass of wine helped.

1   Do you think Lalita is a member of a 'special population'? If so, in what way?
2   What are the considerations for Lalita with her medications?
3   Lalita appears to have a busy life – what questions might you wish to ask Lalita to help her work out why she is feeling as she is? What specifically might you want to clarify?
4   What advice might you give Lalita around her medicines and the issues specific to her?

IF I REMEMBER 5 THINGS FROM THIS CHAPTER:

1   A large proportion of the population could be considered as being in a special group with medicines management.
2   People may have more than one additional consideration.
3   Drug dosages may need to be altered depending on renal or liver function.
4   Person-centred medicines optimisation is key to ensuring the most effective dose.
5   Lifestyle factors must also be considered for medicines optimisation.

ANSWERS TO CASE STUDY QUESTIONS

1   Lalita is a woman from Bangladesh and of Asian origin, and she is also overweight. Her ethnicity and family history make her a special population with regards to hypertension but also for considerations of her medications. Amlodipine (a calcium channel blocker) has been known to have a slightly higher bioavailability in females compared to men due to body composition and weight. Hypertension is more prevalent in Asian women due to lifestyle factors, diet (sodium) and also stress. Her continued paracetamol and alcohol intake may be a contributing factor too.
2   The cautions link to her position as 'special' with considerations of her lifestyle, age, gender, stress levels, ethnicity and family history. If she is perimenopausal, this may have led to some of the problems she mentioned, so look at her pattern of taking her

amlodipine to minimise daytime tiredness, blood pressure and her level of hydration and alcohol consumption.

3   You might want to clarify:

- o   Whether the level of stress is a concern and what means she has to manage or control it.
- o   What she is specifically worried about and her support networks.
- o   How she takes her medication – this may be linked with food stuffs (e.g. grapefruit or citrus juice or sodium).
- o   Due to her body mass index explore if she has signs of diabetes mellitus and the link with renal clearance and medications.
- o   Explore her alcohol intake.
- o   Her use of paracetamol and the amount she takes on a daily/weekly basis.
- o   Her menstrual history and why she thinks she is premenopausal and implications for her hormone levels and the symptoms.
- o   Whether she might be pregnant.

4   You might want to give Lalita advice on the following:

- o   Stress management and her support network plus other services in school for her son.
- o   Guidance on how to take amlodipine and other drug or food interactions.
- o   Guidance on frequency of paracetamol use and rebound headaches.
- o   Guidance if needed on safe alcohol intake and spotting problem drinking.
- o   If she might be pregnant consideration of which drugs are safe in pregnancy.

REFERENCES AND RECOMMENDED READING

Age UK (2017) More harm than good. Available at: www.ageuk.org.uk/globalassets/age-uk/documents/reports-and-publications/reports-and-briefings/health--wellbeing/medication/190819_more_harm_than_good.pdf

British Medical Association and Royal Pharmaceutical Society (2022) *British National Formulary 83*. London: BMJ Group and Pharmaceutical Press.

Bruno, C.D., Harmatz, J.S., Duan, S.X., Zhang, Q., Chow, C.R. and Greenblatt, D.J. (2021) Effect of lipophilicity on drug distribution and elimination: Influence of obesity. *British Journal of Clinical Pharmacology*, 87: 3197–3205.

Chu, T. (2014) Gender differences in pharmacokinetics. Available at: www.medscape.com/viewarticle/833946_5

Farrukh, F., Abbasi, A., Jawed, M., Almas, A., Jafar, T., Virani, S.S. and Samad, Z. (2022) Hypertension in women: A South-Asian perspective. *Frontiers in Cardiovascular Medicine*, 9: 880374. doi:10.3389/fcvm.2022.880374.

Grimsrud, K.N., Sherwin, C.M.T., Constance, J.E., Tak, C., Zuppa, A.F., Spigarelli, M.G. and Mihalopoulos, N.L. (2015) Special population considerations and regulatory affairs for clinical research. *Clinical Research and Regulatory Affairs*, 32(2), 45–54. https://doi.org/10.3109/10601333.2015.1001900

Hunter, H.K., Gildengorin, G., Karliner, L., Fontil, V., Pramanik, R. and Potter, M.B. (2022) Differences in hypertension medication prescribing for Black Americans and their association with hypertension outcomes. *The Journal of the American Board of Family Medicine*, 35(1): 26–34. doi:10.3122/jabfm.2022.01.210276.

Izzo, A.A. (2012) *Interactions between Herbs and Conventional Drugs: Overview of the Clinical Data*, Medical principles and practice, 21(5): 404–428. https://doi.org/10.1159/000334488.

Joint Formulary Committee (2024) British National Formulary. Available at: https://bnf.nice.org.uk/

Koopmans, A.B., Braakman, M.H., Vinkers, D.J., Hoek, H.W. and van Harten, P.N. (2021) Meta-analysis of probability estimates of worldwide variation of CYP2D6 and CYP2C19. *Transl Psychiatry*, *11*, 141. https://doi.org/10.1038/s41398-020-01129-1

Latif, A., Faull, C., Ali, A., Wilson, E., Caswell, G., Anderson, C. and Pollock, K. (2020) Caring for palliative care patients at home: Medicines management principles and considerations. *The Pharmaceutical Journal Online*: doi:10.1211/PJ.2020.20207954.

National Institute for Health and Care Excellence (NICE) (2022a) Hypertension in adults: Diagnosis and management. Available at: www.nice.org.uk/guidance/ng136/chapter/Recommendations#choosing-antihypertensive-drug-treatment-for-people-with-or-without-type-2-diabetes

National Institute for Health and Care Excellence (NICE) (2022b) Obesity: Identification, assessment and management. Available at: www.nice.org.uk/guidance/cg189/chapter/Recommendations#pharmacological-interventions

National Institute for Health and Care Excellence (NICE) (2015) Care of dying adults in the last days of life. NICE guideline [NG31]. Available at: www.nice.org.uk/guidance/ng31

NHS England (2016) Stopping over medication of people with a learning disability, autism or both (STOMP). Available at: www.england.nhs.uk/learning-disabilities/improving-health/stomp

Olafuyi, O., Parekh, N., Wright, J. and Koenig, J. (2021) Inter-ethnic differences in pharmacokinetics – is there more that unites than divides? *Pharmacology Research and Perspectives*, *9*(6): e00890. https://doi.org/10.1002/prp2.890

Royal Pharmaceutical Society (2016) How can you encourage medicines optimisation for people with a learning disability? Available at: www.rpharms.com/Portals/0/RPS%20document%20library/Open%20access/Policy/learning-disability-mo-article-160324.pdf

Sinnott, S-J., Douglas, I.J., Smeeth, L., Williamson, E. and Tomlinson, L.A. (2020) First line drug treatment for hypertension and reductions in blood pressure according to age and ethnicity: Cohort study in UK primary care. *BMJ*, 371: m4080. doi:10.1136/bmj.m4080.

Smit, C., De Hoogd, S., Brüggemann, R.J.M. and Knibbe, C.A.J. (2018) Obesity and drug pharmacology: A review of the influence of obesity on pharmacokinetic and pharmacodynamic parameters. *Expert Opinion on Drug Metabolism & Toxicology*, *14*(3): 275–285. doi:10.1080/17425255.2018.1440287.

Streetman, D.S. (2017) Pharmacogenomics and race: Can heritage affect drug disposition? Available at: www.wolterskluwer.com/en/expert-insights/pharmacogenomics-and-race-can-heritage-affect-drug-disposition

Tchang, B.G., Aras, M., Kumar, R.B. and Aronne, L.J. (2021) Pharmacologic treatment of overweight and obesity in adults. In K.R. Feingold, B. Anawalt, M.R. Blackman, et al. (eds), *Endotext*. South Dartmouth, MA: MDText.com, Inc. Available at: www.ncbi.nlm.nih.gov/books/NBK279038/

US Food and Drug Administration (2018) Questions and answers: Risk of next-morning impairment after use of insomnia drugs; FDA requires lower recommended doses for certain drugs containing zolpidem (Ambien, Ambien CR, Edluar, and Zolpimist). Available at: www.fda.gov/drugs/drug-safety-and-availability/questions-and-answers-risk-next-morning-impairment-after-use-insomnia-drugs-fda-requires-lower

Watson, M., Armstrong, P., Gannon, C., Sykes, N. and Black, I. (2023) Palliative care adult network guidelines plus. Available at: https://book.pallcare.info

Whittaker, C.F., Miklich, M.A., Patel, R.S. and Fink, J.C. (2018) Medication safety principles and practice in CKD. *Clinical Journal of the American Society of Nephrology: CJASN*, 13(11), 1738–1746. https://doi.org/10.2215/CJN.00580118

Willacy, H. (2022) Drug prescribing in renal impairment. Available at: https://patient.info/doctor/drug-prescribing-in-renal-impairment

Wood, S., Petty, D., Glidewell, L. and Raynor, D.K.T. (2018) Application of prescribing recommendations in older people with reduced kidney function: A cross-sectional study in general practice. *British Journal of General Practice*, 68(670): e378–e387 https://bjgp.org/content/68/670/e378.long

APPENDIX: DRUG CONVERSION TABLES AND CALCULATION FORMULAS

CONVERSION BETWEEN UNITS

Weights

Kilograms (kg) to grams (g) multiply (×) by 1000

Grams (g) to milligrams (mg) multiply (×) by 1000

Milligrams (mg) to micrograms (mcg) multiply (×) by 1000

Grams (g) to kilograms (kg) divide (÷) by 1000

Milligrams (mg) to grams (g) divide (÷) by 1000

Micrograms (mcg) to milligrams (mg) divide (÷) by 1000

Liquids

Litres (l) to millilitres (ml) multiply (×) by 1000

Decilitres (dl) to millilitres (ml) multiply (×) by 100

Centilitres (cl) to millilitres (ml) multiply (×) by 10

millilitres (ml) to litres (l) divide (÷) by 1000

millilitres (ml) to decilitres (dl) divide (÷) by 100

millilitres (ml) to centilitres (cl) divide (÷) by 10

USEFUL FORMULAS

Tablets or capsules

$$\text{Number of tablets/capsules} = \frac{\textit{what you want (dose prescribed)}}{\textit{what you have (stock dose)}}$$

Liquid medicines or injections

$$\text{Volume to be give (mls)} = \frac{\textit{what you want (dose prescribed)}}{\textit{what you have (stock dose)}} \times \textit{what volume it is in (mls)}$$

Drug calculations based on body weight

$$\text{Dose to be given} = \text{dose per kg} \times \text{body weight (kg)}$$

Calculating body surface area

$$\text{Body surface area} \left(m^2\right) = \sqrt{\frac{\text{weight (kg)} \times \text{height (cm)}}{3600}}$$

Flow rates using infusion pumps

$$\text{Rate (ml / hr)} = \frac{\textit{volume to be infused (ml)}}{\textit{duration of infusion (hours)}}$$

Calculate rate/hour of a fixed delivery dose of a medication

$$\text{Rate (ml / hr)} = \frac{\textit{hourly dose (mg per ml)}}{\textit{concentration of stock (mg per ml)}}$$

Calculate the concentration of a solution

$$\text{Concentration of stock (mg / ml)} = \frac{\textit{stock strength (mg)}}{\textit{volume of stock solution (ml)}}$$

GLOSSARY

Agonist: a substance that binds to a receptor to produce a response

Antagonist: a substance that binds to a receptor to stop a response

Antibiotic resistance: bacteria that become resistant to antibiotics. This is a natural process in excess exposure to antibiotics. Examples include: methicillin-resistant *Staphylococcus aureus* or vancomycin-resistant *Enterococcus*

Apoptosis: normal programmed cell death to remove old or unwanted cells in the body

Arrythmia: abnormal heart rhythm

Blood brain barrier: a semipermeable barrier of endothelial cells that stop pathogens, larger molecules and some drugs from entering the central nervous system

Bronchospasm: constriction of the muscles in the bronchi of the lungs reducing air entry

Cytochrome P450 (CYP): these are a group of enzymes that are involved in the metabolism of drugs, mainly in the liver. There are more than 50 known CYP450 enzymes but CYP1A2, CYP2C9, CYP2C19, CYP2D6, CYP3A4 and CYP3A5 enzymes metabolise 90% of drugs. Many drug interactions occur because a drug either inhibits or enhances the effects of a CYP enzyme. Genetic variations can occur which affect the expression of genes that code for these enzymes which then affect how people react to the drug (see Chapter 9)

Cytokines: small proteins that are released by cells and act as messengers between cells, particularly in the immune system

Cytotoxic: kills cells

Gastric resistant: avoids being broken down in the stomach

Half-life: time taken for half the drug to be removed from the body

Hypercholesterolaemia: high blood cholesterol

Hyperkalaemia: high blood potassium – increases risk of cardiac arrythmias

Hypertension: high blood pressure

Hypertensive crisis: a sudden, severe, uncontrolled increase in blood pressure

Hypoglycaemia: low blood sugar

Hypokalaemia: low blood potassium

Immunosuppression: a weakened immune system

Inflammation: part of the body's innate protective defence system which has five cardinal signs: redness, heat, pain, swelling, loss of function

Inhibitor: a chemical or drug that interferes with the action of another substance such as an enzyme

Interleukins: a form of cytokine

Lymphocytes: white blood cells

Modified release: release of drugs is delayed, prolonged or certain amounts are released at a time

Myelosuppression: bone marrow suppression resulting in the production of fewer red blood cells, white blood cells and platelets

Nephrotoxic: poisoning or damaging the kidneys

Neurotransmitter: a chemical messenger that is released from nerve cells to allow signals between nerve cells

Nociceptive pain: refers to the normal response to noxious insult or injury of tissues such as skin, muscles, visceral organs, joints, tendons or bones

Osteoclasts: cells that break down bone

QT prolongation: an increase in the time when the electrical activity in the ventricle of heart returns to the resting state. This can result in abnormal heart rhythms, especially Torsardes de Pointes, a ventricular tachycardia where the height of the QRS complex on an ECG gets bigger and smaller; this can lead to sudden death

Receptor: a protein that binds a specific substance to cause a response

SSRIs: selective serotonin reuptake inhibitors, a form of antidepressant

T cells: a type of white blood cell (T lymphocyte)

Thromboembolism: a blood clot that originates from another part of the body

Tissue necrosis factor (TNF): a cytokine that can help regulate inflammation and signal to cells that can kill cancer cells

Topical: applied onto a part of the body

Transdermal: through the skin

Ventricular arrythmias: abnormal heart rhythms originating from the ventricles of the heart

INDEX

Page numbers in **bold** indicate tables and in *italic* indicate figures.

nadolol, 144
naproxen, 189, 191
naratriptan, 221
nasal congestion, 211–12
natalizumab, 108
nausea and vomiting, 228–32, 233
nebivolol, 147–8
neuralgia, **184**
neuritis, **184**
neuropathic pain, 183, *183*, 186
neuroprotective drugs, 110
nicardipine hydrochloride, 142
nifedipine, 133, 142
nitrates, 134, 150–1
nitrofurantoin, 46
nociception, 182, 183, **184**
nociceptive pain, 183, *183*
non-adherence *see* medication adherence/
    non-adherence
non-nociceptive pain, 183, *183*, 186
non-steroidal antiinflammatory drugs
    (NSAIDs), 6, 188–94, 221
  in analgesic ladder, *185*
  for blood clotting, 167, 168, 179
  in compound preparations, 195
  in pregnancy and breastfeeding, 42, 179, 205
nystatin, 55–6

obesity, 243
ocrelizumab, 108–9
oestrogens, 112
ofatumumab, 109
olmesartan medoxomil, 139
olodaterol, 19, **25**
omeprazole, 218–19
opicapone, 97
opioids, 197–203
  in analgesic ladder, 185, *185*
  cautions, 185–6, 187, 205
  in compound preparations, 194–6
  ethnicity and, 242–3
  for haemorrhoids, 215–16
  in pregnancy and breastfeeding, 205
orlistat, 244
orphenadrine hydrochloride, 95
oseltamivir, 58
osmotic diuretics, 155
osmotic laxatives, 224, 226
osteoporosis, 93, 112–17
  bisphosphonates, 113–16, 128, 242
  bone reabsorption inhibitors, 113, 116, 117
  monoclonal antibodies, 113, 117, 128
  parathyroid hormones and analogues, 113,
    116–17
over-the-counter (OTC) medicines, 1, 3, 5, 6,
    185, 189, 195, 208–9
  see also common symptoms

oxycodone, 194, 199
ozanimod, 103, 106–7, 127

pain, 182–206
  analgesic ladder, 184–5, *185*
  case study, 205, 206
  cautions with analgesia, 185–6, 187, 205
  compound analgesic preparations, 194–6
  definitions and overview, 182–4, *183*, **184**
    acute pain, 183
    chronic pain, 183
    inflammatory pain, 183, *183*
    neuropathic pain, 183, *183*, 186
    nociceptive pain, 183, *183*
  headaches, 183, 186, 220–4
    cluster headaches, 186, 203–4, 221
    medication overuse headaches, 187,
      204, 221
    migraine, 183, 186, 203–4, 221–4, 233
    sinus headaches, 221
    tension headaches, 220
  non-pharmacological approaches, 186
  non-steroidal antiinflammatory drugs
    (NSAIDs), 6, 188–94, 221
    in analgesic ladder, *185*
    for blood clotting, 167, 168, 179
    in compound preparations, 195
    in pregnancy and breastfeeding, 42,
      179, 205
  opioids, 197–203
    in analgesic ladder, 185, *185*
    cautions, 185–6, 187, 205
    in compound preparations, 194–6
    ethnicity and, 242–3
    for haemorrhoids, 215–16
    in pregnancy and breastfeeding, 205
  paracetamol, 184, 187–8
    in analgesic ladder, *185*
    cautions, 185, 205
    in compound preparations, 195–6
    in pregnancy and breastfeeding, 205
  in pregnancy and breastfeeding, 205
pain threshold, **184**
pain tolerance level, **184**
palliative care, 241–2
paracetamol, 184, 187–8
  in analgesic ladder, *185*
  cautions, 185, 205
  in compound preparations
    dihydrocodeine with paracetamol,
      195, 196
    paracetamol with codeine, 195–6
    tramadol with paracetamol, 195, 196
  in pregnancy and breastfeeding, 205
parasympathomimetics, 119, 123
parathyroid hormones and analogues, 113,
    116–17